Midface and Periocular Rejuvenation

Editor

ANTHONY P. SCLAFANI

FACIAL PLASTIC SURGERY CLINICS OF NORTH AMERICA

www.facialplastic.theclinics.com

Consulting Editor
J. REGAN THOMAS

May 2015 • Volume 23 • Number 2

ELSEVIER

1600 John F. Kennedy Boulevard • Suite 1800 • Philadelphia, Pennsylvania, 19103-2899

http://www.theclinics.com

FACIAL PLASTIC SURGERY CLINICS OF NORTH AMERICA Volume 23, Number 2
May 2015 ISSN 1064-7406, ISBN-13: 978-0-323-37595-5

Editor: Joanne Husovski
Developmental Editor: Susan Showalter

Facial Plastic Surgery Clinics of North America (ISSN 1064-7406) is published quarterly by Elsevier Inc., 360 Park Avenue South, New York, NY 10010-1710. Months of issue are February, May, August, and November. Business and Editorial Offices: 1600 John F. Kennedy Blvd., Suite 1800, Philadelphia, PA 19103-2899. Periodicals postage paid at New York, NY, and additional mailing offices. Subscription prices are $390.00 per year (US individuals), $525.00 per year (US institutions), $445.00 per year (Canadian individuals), $653.00 per year (Canadian institutions), $535.00 per year (foreign individuals), $653.00 per year (foreign institutions), $185.00 per year (US students), and $255.00 per year (foreign students). Foreign air speed delivery is included in all *Clinics* subscription prices. All prices are subject to change without notice. POSTMASTER: Send address changes to *Facial Plastic Surgery Clinics*, Elsevier Health Sciences Division, Subscription Customer Service, 3251 Riverport Lane, Maryland Heights, MO 63043. **Customer service: 1-800-654-2452 (US and Canada); 1-314-447-8871 (outside US and Canada); Fax: 314-447-8029; E-mail:** journalscustomerservice-usa@elsevier.com **(for print support);** journalsonline support-usa@elsevier.com **(for online support).**

Reprints. For copies of 100 or more of articles in this publication, please contact the Commercial Reprints Department, Elsevier Inc., 360 Park Avenue South, New York, NY 10010-1710. Tel.: 212-633-3874; Fax: 212-633-3820; E-mail: reprints@elsevier.com.

Facial Plastic Surgery Clinics of North America is covered in *MEDLINE/PubMed* (*Index Medicus*).

Contributors

CONSULTING EDITOR

J. REGAN THOMAS, MD
Mansueto Professor and Chairman,
Department of Otolaryngology–Head and Neck
Surgery, University of Illinois at Chicago,
Chicago, Illinois

EDITOR

ANTHONY P. SCLAFANI, MD, FACS
Surgeon Director and Director of Facial Plastic
Surgery, The New York Eye and Ear Infirmary of
Mount Sinai, Professor of Otolaryngology,
Icahn School of Medicine at Mount Sinai,
New York, New York

AUTHORS

GREGORY BRANHAM, MD
Chief, Division of Facial Plastic and
Reconstructive Surgery; Professor,
Otolaryngology/Head and Neck Surgery,
Washington University School of Medicine,
St Louis, Missouri

CÉSAR A. BRICEÑO, MD
Assistant Professor, Department of
Ophthalmology and Visual Sciences, Kellogg
Eye Center, University of Michigan, Ann Arbor,
Michigan

JOEL COHEN, MD
AboutSkin Dermatology and DermSurgery,
PC, Englwood, Colorado

JORGE I. DE LA TORRE, MD
Professor and Chief, Division of Plastic
Surgery, University of Alabama at Birmingham;
Staff Surgeon, Birmingham VA Medical Center,
Birmingham, Alabama

GREGORY DIBELIUS, MD
Resident, Department of Otolaryngology–Head
and Neck Surgery, The New York Eye and Ear
Infirmary of Mount Sinai, New York, New York

ROBERT D. ENGLE, MD
Division of Otolaryngology and Head-Neck
Surgery, Department of Surgery, Albany
Medical College, Albany, New York

BENJAMIN P. ERICKSON, MD
Bascom Palmer Eye Institute, University of
Miami Miller School of Medicine, Miami, Florida

MARK J. GLASGOLD, MD
Clinical Associate Professor, Department of
Surgery, Robert Wood Johnson Medical
School, Rutgers University, New Brunswick,
New Jersey; Private Practice, Highland Park,
New Jersey

ROBERT A. GLASGOLD, MD
Clinical Assistant Professor, Department of
Surgery, Robert Wood Johnson Medical
School, Rutgers University, New Brunswick,
New Jersey; Private Practice, Highland Park,
New Jersey

LISA D. GRUNEBAUM, MD
Assistant Professor, Division of Facial Plastic
and Reconstructive Surgery, Department of
Otolaryngology and Dermatology, University of
Miami Miller School of Medicine, Miami, Florida

MEIR HERSHCOVITCH, MD
Mittelman Plastic Surgery, Los Altos, California

JOHN B. HOLDS, MD, FACS
Clinical Professor, Ophthalmology and
Otolaryngology/Head and Neck Surgery,
Saint Louis University, St Louis, Missouri

THEDA C. KONTIS, MD
Assistant Professor, Department of
Otolaryngology–Head and Neck Surgery,
Johns Hopkins Medical Institutions, Baltimore,
Maryland

SAMUEL M. LAM, MD, FACS
Director, Willow Bend Wellness Center,
Plano, Texas

WENDY W. LEE, MD
Associate Professor of Clinical Ophthalmology
and Dermatology Oculofacial Plastic and
Reconstructive Surgery, Orbit and Oncology,
Bascom Palmer Eye Institute, University of
Miami Miller School of Medicine, Miami, Florida

ANDRE YUAN LEVESQUE, MD
Assistant Professor, Division of Plastic
Surgery, University of Alabama at Birmingham,
Birmingham, Alabama

GUY G. MASSRY, MD
Clinical Professor of Ophthalmology,
Ophthalmic Plastic and Reconstructive
Surgery, Keck School of Medicine, University
of Southern California, Beverly Hills, California

HARRY MITTELMAN, MD
Fellow, American Academy of Facial Plastic
and Reconstructive Surgery, Mittelman Plastic
Surgery, Los Altos, California

PAUL S. NASSIF, MD
Facial Plastic Surgery, Nassif MD Plastic
Surgery, Beverly Hills, California; Assistant
Clinical Professor, Division of Facial Plastic and
Reconstructive Surgery, Department of
Otolaryngology – Head and Neck Surgery,
Keck School of Medicine University of
Southern California, Los Angeles, California

STEPHEN W. PERKINS, MD
Meridian Plastic Surgeons; Associate Clinical
Professor, Department of Otolaryngology/
Head and Neck Surgery, Indiana University
School of Medicine, Indianapolis, Indiana

TAYLOR R. POLLEI, MD
Division of Otolaryngology and Head-Neck
Surgery, Department of Surgery, Albany
Medical College, Albany, New York; Williams
Center Plastic Surgery Specialists, Department
of Facial Plastic and Reconstructive Surgery,
Williams Center for Excellence, Latham,
New York

LESLEY A. RABACH, MD
Private Practice, New York, New York

ANTHONY P. SCLAFANI, MD, FACS
Surgeon Director and Director of Facial
Plastic Surgery, The New York Eye and Ear
Infirmary of Mount Sinai; Professor of
Otolaryngology, Icahn School of Medicine at
Mount Sinai, New York, New York

SCOTT SHADFAR, MD
Meridian Plastic Surgeons, Indianapolis,
Indiana

WILLIAM E. SILVER, MD
Clinical Instructor, Department of
Otolaryngology, Head and Neck Surgery,
Emory University; Private Practice, Premier
Image Cosmetic and Laser Surgery, Atlanta,
Georgia

DANNY J. SOARES, MD
Private Practice, Mesos Plastic and Laser
Surgery, Lady Lake, Florida

MARIETTA TAN, MD
Resident, Department of Otolaryngology–Head
and Neck Surgery, Johns Hopkins University
School of Medicine, Baltimore, Maryland

SATYEN UNDAVIA, MD
Private Practice, Head and Neck Associates,
Havertown, Philadelphia

EDWIN F. WILLIAMS III, MD, FACS
Division of Otolaryngology and Head-Neck
Surgery, Department of Surgery, Albany
Medical College, Albany, New York; Williams
Center Plastic Surgery Specialists, Department
of Facial Plastic and Reconstructive Surgery,
Williams Center for Excellence, Latham,
New York

DONALD B. YOO, MD
Facial Plastic Surgery, Nassif MD Plastic Surgery, Beverly Hills, California; Assistant Clinical Professor, Division of Facial Plastic and Reconstructive Surgery, Department of Otolaryngology – Head and Neck Surgery, Keck School of Medicine University of Southern California, Los Angeles, California; Assistant Clinical Professor, Division of Facial Plastic and Reconstructive Surgery, Department of Otolaryngology – Head and Neck Surgery, David Geffen School of Medicine at the University of California, Los Angeles, California

SANDY X. ZHANG-NUNES, MD
Assistant Professor, Department of Ophthalmology, USC Eye Institute, Keck School of Medicine, University of Southern California Keck School of Medicine, Los Angeles, California

Contents

The upper eyelid serves the important anatomic function of protecting the eye and rewetting the cornea to maintain vision. The complex dynamic action of the upper eyelid explains its relatively complex anatomy. The brow has an important supportive role. Studies have revealed facial characteristics perceived as youthful and aged, and the anatomic basis of these changes is defined at many levels. Characteristic aging changes in the upper eyelid and brow create an appearance of aging and opportunities for functional and aesthetic improvement.

This article reviews the key anatomic structures in the region of the midface, including important surface and bony landmarks, innervation, blood supply, muscle layers, and fat compartments. It also discusses changes in these structures related to the aging process and aesthetic analysis of the midface to aid with operative planning.

 Video of (1) External Browpexy Procedure, (2) Nasal Fat Preservation, (3) Nasal Fat Preservation: Orbitoglabellar Groove, (4) Lacrimal Gland Repositioning, and (5) Brassiere Suture Fixation of Brow Fat Pad accompanyies this article

A variety of surgical adjuncts can be added to upper eyelid blepharoplasty with the goal of enhancing surgical results and patient satisfaction. All of these procedures are minimally invasive and most are performed through a standard eyelid crease incision. These procedures can be added to stabilize or conservatively lift the outer brow, prevent the stigmata of postoperative volume loss, improve the brow-eyelid transition and contour, and reposition a prolapsed lacrimal gland. The procedures are generally straightforward, easily learned, and complication free. Familiarity with these techniques provides the aesthetic eyelid surgeon with added options to improve surgical results.

Eyebrow and upper eyelid aging occurs in all tissue planes, and manifests most commonly in skin quality, tissue volume loss (soft tissue and bone), and tissue descent. All these involutional changes are amenable to less-invasive (nonsurgical) interventions with natural and aesthetically pleasing results. It is critical for aesthetic facial surgeons to familiarize themselves with these procedures because they are in high demand by patients. This article outlines current concepts of nonsurgical management options for brow and upper eyelid aging. The anatomy and age-related changes in these structures are reviewed, and minimally invasive techniques to address these changes are detailed.

Surgical management of the aging upper face has taken on a critical role in total facial rejuvenation, with a variety of techniques available. The hallmarks of the aging upper third of the face and periorbital region most commonly manifest as rhytids, brow descent, prolapse of periorbital fat, dermatochalasis, and volume loss and hollowing. The surrounding structures should be assessed individually and their relationships carefully analyzed to guide selection of the appropriate treatment. In this article, the authors explore the various approaches and techniques available for rejuvenation of the upper face, including the upper periorbital region.

 A video of midface skeletal enhancement accompanies this article

Alloplastic malar augmentation offers a reliable means of achieving a permanent, yet reversible, form of midfacial volume enhancement that serves to correct the changes associated with facial aging, hypoplasia, and congenital malar asymmetry. The degree of augmentation depends on the severity of existing malar bony hypoplasia, soft tissue volume loss/ptosis, or both. Facial aesthetic surgeons have a multitude of implant designs and shapes and implant materials available. The transoral surgical approach with transcutaneous implant suture stabilization is the most commonly used surgical protocol in alloplastic midface augmentation and is, therefore, the technique specifically chosen for review in this article.

No nonsurgical technique can come close to rejuvenating the face like a cervicofacial rhytidectomy. However, one of the most difficult areas to improve during a facelift is the midface. The multi-vector high superficial musculoaponeurotic system (SMAS) facelift and extended lower-lid midface lift are important techniques that can adequately address the midface during rhytidectomy. The multi-vector high SMAS facelift is a natural extension of a traditional SMAS plication or imbrication facelift. The extended lower-lid midface lift can be an important adjunct during a facelift or as an independent procedure to address the midface.

Early facial rejuvenation focused largely on the upper and lower thirds of the face. More recently, improvements in understanding of midfacial aging and anatomy have paralleled the development of endoscopic and minimally invasive surgical techniques. The midface is now understood to include both the lower lid subunit and the cheek down to the nasolabial fold. Many surgical techniques for midface rejuvenation have been used, including skin tightening with direct excision, skin–muscle flaps, isolated fat pad transposition, and subperiosteal lifting. The methods of endoscopic subperiosteal midface lifting and endoscopic malar fat pad lifting are discussed.

 A video of transpalpebral midface rejuvenation accompanies this article

Aging of the midface is a complex aesthetic problem requiring an individualized and multifaceted surgical approach. The objective of harmonious rejuvenation of the entire face as well as increasing patient interest in midface rejuvenation mandates surgical familiarity with these techniques. Midface rejuvenation procedures have evolved from traditional laterally based rhytidectomy techniques with superolateral elevation to modern centrofacial approaches designed to achieve more vertical vectors of elevation. These approaches are informed by an evolving understanding of the multiple processes that contribute to the aged appearance of the midface and are based on lower blepharoplasty surgical techniques.

There is currently a major paradigm shift from excision-based surgery to strictly volume enhancement. Because there is still no perfect facial filler, development of synthetic facial injectables continue to advance at a remarkable pace. Each type of filler carries a specific characteristic that makes it more suitable for a certain clinical application. The continuing change in facial fillers offers the possibility for volume augmentation procedures with less downtime and without the need for harvesting fat. We predict that volume enhancement will continue to play an increasing role as both a complementary and as a stand-alone procedure in facial rejuvenation.

The aging midface has long been overlooked in cosmetic surgery. Our understanding of facial aging in terms of 3 dimensions has placed increased importance on volume restoration. Although an "off-label" indication for most fillers in this facial region, volumization of the midface with injectable fillers is usually a safe and straightforward procedure technically. Injectors, nevertheless, need to have an excellent understanding of facial anatomy and the characteristics of the injected products should problems arise.

 Videos of female and male glabellar injections and lateral canthal line injection accompany this article

Initially popularized for the treatment of strabismus and blepharospasm, injection of botulinum neurotoxin has become the most commonly performed cosmetic treatment in the United States. Injection techniques have been particularly well-studied in the midface and periocular region, and patient satisfaction tends to be very high. We review the salient differences among available neurotoxins, how to optimally reconstitute them, how to inject the forehead, glabella, lateral canthal lines ("crow's feet"), infralid region, and transverse nasal lines ("bunny lines"), how to sculpt the brow, and how to manage potential complications.

The eyes play a central role in the perception of facial beauty. The goal of periorbital rejuvenation surgery is to restore youthful proportions and focus attention on the eyes. Blepharoplasty is the third most common cosmetic procedure performed today. Because of the attention placed on the periorbital region, preventing and managing complications is important. Obtaining a thorough preoperative history and physical examination can significantly reduce the incidence of many of the complications. This article focuses on the preoperative evaluation as it relates to preventable complications, followed by common intraoperative and postoperative complications and their management.

FACIAL PLASTIC SURGERY CLINICS OF NORTH AMERICA

DOWNLOAD Free App!

Review Articles
THE CLINICS

NOW AVAILABLE FOR YOUR iPhone and iPad

Preface
Midface and Periocular Rejuvenation

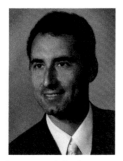

Anthony P. Sclafani, MD, FACS
Editor

It is with great pleasure that I introduce this issue of *Facial Plastic Surgery Clinics of North America*, dedicated to the esthetic treatment of the midface and periorbital regions. The authors in this issue are world-renowned leaders in the field and present their topics on a strong foundation of anatomy and physiology of these areas. From minimally invasive techniques to soft tissue treatments and skeletal modifications, these authors present a comprehensive view of cosmetic surgery of the midface and orbital areas. The more recent concepts of midfacial volume augmentation with autologous fat and injectable fillers, as well as esthetic contouring of the face with neurotoxins, are discussed. Finally, management, and more importantly, avoidance of complications are presented.

I hope you enjoy reading this issue of *Facial Plastic Surgery Clinics of North America* as much as I did, it strengthens your understanding of the anatomy, physiology, and chronopathology of the midface and periorbita, and allows you to more confidently perform minimally invasive and surgical management of these areas.

Anthony P. Sclafani, MD, FACS
Icahn School of Medicine at Mt. Sinai
Facial Plastic Surgery
The New York Eye and
Ear Infirmary of Mt. Sinai
310 East 14th Street
New York, NY 10003, USA

E-mail address:
asclafani@nyee.edu

Facial Plast Surg Clin N Am 23 (2015) xiii
http://dx.doi.org/10.1016/j.fsc.2015.02.001
1064-7406/15/$ – see front matter © 2015 Published by Elsevier Inc.

Brow/Upper Lid Anatomy, Aging and Aesthetic Analysis

 CrossMark

Gregory Branham, MD[a], John B. Holds, MD[b,c],*

KEYWORDS

- Upper eyelid • Brow • Ptosis • Blepharoplasty • Browlift • Dermatochalasis • Blepharochalasis

KEY POINTS

- The complex anatomy of the eyelid and inter-relation of the eyelid–eyebrow continuum have important functional and cosmetic consequences in the periorbital region.
- A study of what is considered attractive, youthful, or aesthetically desirable is useful in patient evaluation and defining surgical goals.
- Characteristic aging changes in the central face have a definable anatomic basis and cosmetic consequences amenable to surgical correction.

BROW AND UPPER EYELID ANATOMY

The eyebrow and upper eyelid comprise the periorbital area. In considering rejuvenation of the aging face, this zone is evaluated and treated as a single area, because there is an intricate interaction between the eyebrows and the upper eyelid in the aging process. This intricate and interdependent relationship extends into the forehead and frontalis muscle in a relationship defined by Hering law.[1] The periorbital region is bounded superiorly by the forehead and laterally by the temporal region. They meet centrally at the glabellar region. Lower eyelid anatomy, aging, and surgical treatment are covered elsewhere in this issue.

EYEBROW SOFT TISSUE

The eyebrow is comprised of the skin and soft tissues that cover the superior orbital rim. Visually it is demarcated superiorly by the first forehead crease that curves above the hair bearing brow skin. Inferiorly the subciliary brow ends at the arcus marginalis on the superior orbital rim, transitioning to the upper eyelid. The upper eyelid extends inferiorly to the upper lid margin inferiorly apposing the globe (**Fig. 1**).

The eyebrow skin contains specialized hair follicles that define the brow. These hair follicles are different from other follicles in their orientation and growth cycle. Unlike hair follicles of the scalp, the brow cilia have a limited growth pattern and can be permanently injured with plucking or shaving. Once lost, the brow cilia are difficult to recreate with grafting. Deep to the hair-bearing skin of the brow is the corrugator supercilii muscle (**Fig. 2**), which originates from the superior orbital rim at the medial end of the brow and runs along the superior orbital ridge for a variable distance to terminate at the lateral third of the brow. The corrugator muscle inserts into the brow skin and is responsible for the vertical lines in the glabellar region perpendicular to its orientation.

The authors have no current disclosures.

[a] Division of Facial Plastic and Reconstructive Surgery, Otolaryngology–Head and Neck Surgery, Department of Otolaryngology, Washington University School of Medicine, 660 South Euclid Avenue, Campus Box 8115, St Louis, MO 63110 USA; [b] Department of Ophthalmology, Saint Louis University, 1755 South Grand Boulevard, St Louis, MO 63104, USA; [c] Department of Otolaryngology/Head and Neck Surgery, Saint Louis University, 3635 Vista Avenue, St Louis, MO 63110, USA

* Corresponding author. Ophthalmic Plastic and Cosmetic Surgery, Inc, 12990 Manchester Road #102, Des Peres, MO 63131.

E-mail address: jholds@sbcglobal.net

facialplastic.theclinics.com

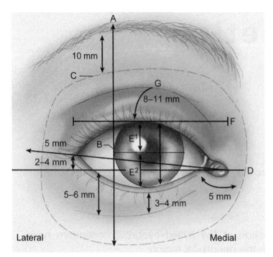

Fig. 1. Topography of the eyelid. (A) The highest point of the brow is at, or lateral to, the lateral limbus. (B) The inferior edge of the brow is shown 10 mm superior to the supraorbital rim. (C) Also shown are ranges for average palpebral height (10–12 mm), width (28–30 mm), (D) and upper lid fold (8–11 mm, with gender and racial differences). Note that the lateral canthus is 2 to 4 mm higher than the medial canthus. (E) Intrapalpebral distance measures 10 to 12 mm. E1, mean reflex distance 1; E2, mean reflex distance 2. (F) Palpebral width. (G) Upper lid fold is 8 to 11 mm. (*From* Most SP, Mobley SR, Larrabee WF Jr. Anatomy of the eyelids [review]. Facial Plast Surg Clin North Am 2005;13:487–92; with permission.)

The procerus muscle lies in the midline of the glabellar region extending inferiorly from the nasion and oriented in a vertical fashion. Contraction of this muscle creates the horizontal lines that appear in the central glabellar region and upper nose. Both the paired corrugator supercilii muscles and the central procerus muscle are strong depressors of the eyebrow.

There is a dense fibrous attachment of the brow to the superior orbital rim that extends inferiorly to the arcus marginalis of the superior orbit. The superior and upper lateral orbital rims complete the osseous boundary of this region.

EYEBROW INNERVATION AND VASCULATURE

Piercing the superior orbital rim through a complete foramen, or traversing through a notch, are the supratrochlear and supraorbital nerves; both are branches of the first division of the trigeminal nerve. The supratrochlear nerve is located approximately 17.5 mm from the midline along the orbital rim. Often a notch can be palpated there. Traversing with the supraorbital nerve is a paired artery and vein of the same name. The supraorbital nerve is located approximately 27.5 mm from the midline along the superior orbital rim. It may traverse through a true foramen or a notch. It also has a paired artery and vein of the same name. These 2 sensory nerves exit the superior orbital rim and

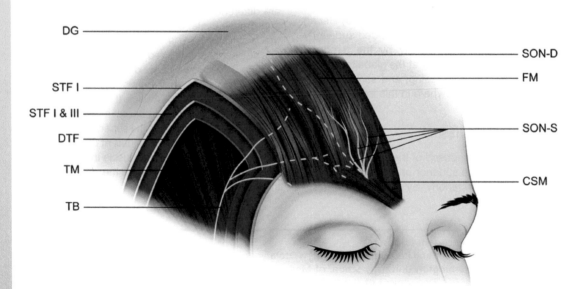

Fig. 2. Fascial layers of the temporal region. CSM, corrugators supercilii muscle; DG, deep galea plane; DTF, deep temporal fascia; FM, frontalis muscle; SON-D, deep division of the supraorbital nerve; SON-S, superficial division of the supraorbital nerve; STF, superficial termporal fascia; STF I, the superficial layer of the temporal fascia; STF II-III, the two deep layers of the superficial temporal fascia; TB, temporal branch of frontal nerve; TM, temporalis muscle. (*From* Lam VB, Czyz CN, Wulc AE. The brow-lid continuum: an anatomic perspective. Clin Plast Surg 2013;40:8; with permission.)

ascend up the forehead, providing sensory innervation to the forehead and scalp to the vertex. The supratrochlear nerve branches medially to provide sensory innervation to the glabellar region and upper lateral nose as well. There is also a small infratrochlear nerve that exits inferior to the supratrochlear nerve and supplies sensation to the side of the nose and medial canthal area.

Motor innervation for the corrugator and procerus muscles is via branches of the upper division of the facial nerve. Lymphatics in this region generally run with the neurovascular bundles and also laterally from the lateral orbital rim.

HERING LAW

Ewald Hering described a symmetric and synergistic relationship of the eye muscles that allowed an individual to track a moving object and to keep that object in focus and fuse images from the 2 eyes. Information from the afferent system provides a symmetric feedback loop to the extraocular musculature that allows this to occur. This same principle applies to the levator superioris and frontalis muscles. If significant dermatochalasis or lid ptosis exists, the levator palpebrae superioris and/or frontalis muscle tone is increased to overcome this inferior displacement of the eyelid.[1] This compensatory hyperactivity of the frontalis muscle is evidenced by increased horizontal forehead rhytids. It is essential to examine the patient with the frontalis muscle relaxed to accurately determine brow position and the presence of lid ptosis. Likewise, when significant brow ptosis is present, it is important to examine the eyelids with the brow in a more youthful elevated position to determine the true extent of the dermatochalasis. Patients are often surprised to see how little dermatochalasis they have when the brow is elevated. Blepharoplasty surgery often unmasks latent lid ptosis or brow ptosis secondary to Hering law. This is because correction of the dermatochalasis diminishes the afferent input to the frontalis and levator muscles, which then relax, revealing the true brow or lid ptosis.

NEUROMODULATORS

It is important to evaluate patients without neuromodulators such as botulinum toxin in effect. Depending on where the botulinum toxin is placed, the brow can be lowered (frontalis muscle injection) or raised (orbital portion of orbicularis oculi). Patients should always be asked about the use of neuromodulators.

EYELID SOFT TISSUE

The function of the upper eyelids is to protect and lubricate the cornea by acting as a barrier to foreign bodies and by restoring the tear film through periodic blinking. Small glands along the lid margin secrete mucous and oil that adds to aqueous lacrimal gland secretion, creating a 3-layer tear film that lubricates the cornea. This tear film breaks down as it is exposed to the air, and the act of blinking restores this delicate balance.

The upper eyelids are composed of several layers (**Fig. 3**). These are typically broken down into the anterior and posterior lamellae. The anterior lamella is comprised of skin and orbicularis muscle. The skin of the eyelids is the thinnest skin of the human body. This provides the necessary flexibility needed for blinking. Because it is

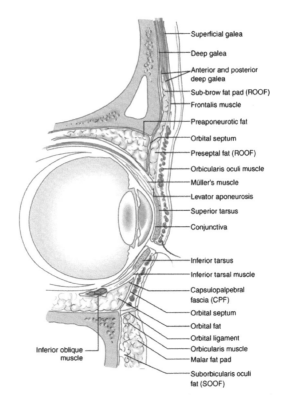

Fig. 3. Cross-sectional anatomy of the upper and lower lids. The capsulopalpebral fascia and inferior tarsal muscle are retractors of the lower lid whereas Müller muscle, the levator muscle, and its aponeurosis are retractors of the upper lid. Note the preseptal positioning of the ROOF and suborbicularis oculi fat. The orbitomalar ligament arises from the arcus marginalis of the inferior orbital rim and inserts on the skin of the lower lid, forming the nasojugal fold. (*From* Most SP, Mobley SR, Larrabee WF Jr. Anatomy of the eyelids [review]. Facial Plast Surg Clin North Am 2005;13:487–92; with permission.)

so thin, it contains few sebaceous glands or adnexal structures. There is also no fat or adipose layer between the skin and the underlying muscles below the preseptal orbicularis. The posterior lamella is composed of the levator muscle and/or levator aponeurosis, Müller muscle, and conjunctiva. Inferiorly, the posterior lamella contains the tarsus instead of the muscle/aponeurosis layer. The tarsus is a specialized dense connective tissue structure that acts as the skeletal support or framework for the eyelid. Within the tarsus are the meibomian glands that secrete mebum, a thick lubricant that contributes the oil layer to the tear film. The lid margin has a tightly adherent mucosal layer that is penetrated by the meibomian ducts. The upper tarsus measures approximately 10 to 12 mm in height at the midpupillary line and tapers medially and laterally. The tarsus is held tightly in position laterally by the upper crus of the lateral canthal tendon, which inserts laterally onto Whitnall tubercle, a bony prominence just inside the orbital rim (**Fig. 4**-G). The medial canthal tendon divides into anterior and posterior divisions that encircle the lacrimal sac. They insert on the anterior and posterior lacrimal crest, respectively. The orbital fat is separated from the posterior lamella by the orbital septum, which is a thin adventitial layer that fuses with the superior edge of the tarsus inferiorly and with the arcus marginalis superiorly.

MUSCULATURE

The orbicularis muscle is a radially oriented muscle that is innervated by the facial nerve and is responsible for the radially oriented crow's feet lines that appear at the lateral canthus over time. The orbicularis muscle has 3 components (**Fig. 5**):

> The orbital portion is the outermost portion of the muscle, and it overlies the superior bony rim and contributes fibers to the cheek, forehead, and temporal region. This portion of the orbicularis is a significant depressor of the eyebrow along with the corrugators and procerus muscles.
>
> The preseptal component lies between the orbital and pretarsal components.
>
> The pretarsal component overlies the tarsus. The preseptal and pretarsal components perform the involuntary blinking function of the eye.

The levator palpebrae superioris arises from the lesser wing of the sphenoid at the orbital apex and is continuous with the levator aponeurosis,

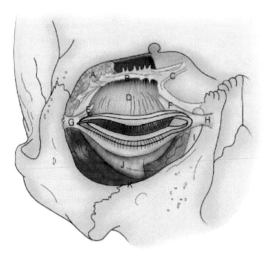

Fig. 4. Tendons and ligaments of the eye. Anatomic diagram of canthal tendons showing attachments of eyelids to anterior orbital connective tissue structures. (A) Orbital lobe of the lacrimal gland, (B) Whitnall' transverse, (C) superior oblique tendon, (D) levator aponeurosis, (E) lateral horn of levator aponeurosis, (F) medial horn of levator aponeurosis, (G) lateral canthal tendon, (H) medial canthal tendon, (I) lacrimal sac, (J) capsulopalpebral fascia, (K) Lockwood suspensory ligament. (*From* Branham GJ. Eyelid and periocular reconstruction. In: Thomas procedures in facial plastic surgery: facial soft tissue reconstruction. Shelton (CT): People's Medical Publishing House-USA; 2011. p. 107; with permission.)

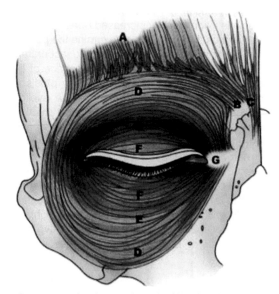

Fig. 5. Periorbital musculature. The orbicularis muscle and adjacent facial muscles. (A) Frontalis. (B) Corrugator supercilii. (C) Procerus, (D) Orbital orbicularis. (E) Preseptal orbicularis. (F) Pretarsal orbicularis. (G) Medial canthal tendon. (*From* Branham GJ. Eyelid and periocular reconstruction. In: Thomas procedures in facial plastic surgery: facial soft tissue reconstruction. Shelton (CT): People's Medical Publishing House-USA; 2011. p. 106; with permission.)

inserting onto the anterior surface of the tarsus (see **Fig. 3**). It is innervated by the superior division of cranial nerve III and serves as the primary elevator of the eyelid. At the posterior surface of the levator aponeurosis and attached to the palpebral conjunctiva, is Müller muscle, innervated by the sympathetic nervous system, which travels via the carotid artery to the ophthalmic vessels and into the muscle. Müller muscle is responsible for 2 to 3 mm of elevation of the upper eyelid as a resting tone and not a voluntary contraction. Disruption of the sympathetic chain along the carotid artery is responsible for Horner syndrome, characterized by lid ptosis, miosis (constricted pupil), and anhydrosis (lack of sweating) of the ipsilateral face.

LACRIMAL SYSTEM

The lacrimal drainage system is comprised of a single punctum at the medial aspect of each upper and lower tarsus, which is connected to a canaliculus that drains into the lacrimal sac, which lies in the lacrimal fossa medially. The lacrimal sac then drains into the nasal cavity by piercing the lateral nasal wall as the nasolacrimal duct and terminating in the interior meatus intranasally. The lacrimal sac, as mentioned earlier, is surrounded by the anterior and posterior limbs of the medial canthal tendon. When blinking occurs, the contraction of the muscle creates tension on the medial canthus and compression of the lacrimal sac that creates a pumping action, thus permitting drainage of the system into the nasal cavity.

ORBITAL FAT COMPARTMENTS

The orbit is considered to have 3 fat compartments in both the upper and lower eyelids (**Fig. 6**). In the upper eyelid, the nasal or medial fat compartment is divided from the central or middle compartment by the superior oblique muscle. The fat is held within the orbit by the orbital septum. The lateral upper eyelid is occupied by the lacrimal gland, which lies in the lacrimal fossa, a bony depression in the superior lateral orbit. Prolapse of the lacrimal gland should not be mistaken for fat and excised.

RETRO-ORBICULARIS OCULI FAT

Beneath the ciliary portion of the brow and associated with the orbital portion of the orbicularis oculi is a fat compartment known as retro-orbicularis oculi fat (ROOF). This fat pad continues into the preseptal portion of the eyelid and is partially

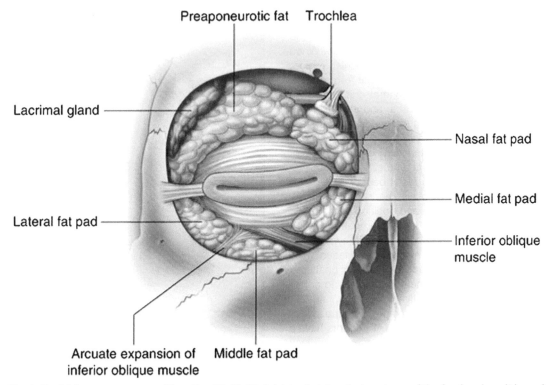

Preaponeurotic fat   Trochlea

Lacrimal gland

Nasal fat pad

Medial fat pad

Lateral fat pad

Inferior oblique muscle

Arcuate expansion of   Middle fat pad
inferior oblique muscle

Fig. 6. Eyelid fat compartments. (*From* Tan KS, Oh SR, Priel A, et al. Surgical anatomy of the forehead, eyelids, and midface for the aesthetic surgeon. In: Massry GG, Murphy MR, Azizzadeh B, editors. Master techniques in blepharoplasty and periorbital rejuvenation. New York: Springer-USA; 2011. p. 16; with permission.)

responsible for the thicker, lower, and less defined eyelid crease seen in the Asian eyelid. Resection of ROOF creates a more sculpted and hollow upper lid and was once felt to be essential to rejuvenate the upper lid/brow complex. This approach has fallen into disfavor, as surgical and aesthetic concepts focus on retaining volume and avoiding the skeletonized, hollowed eye that tends to worsen with age.[2] Often, fullness of the upper lid is an indication that a concomitant brow lift is indicated.

Aging Changes of the Upper Eyelid and Brow Regions

Aesthetic analysis

The eye and adjacent area are instinctively perceived as a central feature of facial beauty. One intuitively looks to the eye to assess age, beauty, health, mood, level of consciousness, and intelligence. Fair or not, these instinctive judgments are wired into the human psyche, and patients wish to modify appearance to alter perception. A study of what is perceived as beautiful in the periocular area along with the anatomic changes of aging will help the surgeon to appropriately assess and advise patients.[3]

Viewing the upper third of the face as an aesthetic unit, the eyebrow and eyelid are considered together in most instances as a continuum.[1] Anatomic changes in the periocular area provide clues to ages from infancy to senescence. When addressing perception of the periocular region, there are several core concepts that form a foundation for beauty. These general characteristics span the borders of age, race, and ethnicity, and include facial symmetry, averageness, and feature size. The casual observer might have difficulty defining these characteristics but instinctively perceives them looking at a face.

Symmetry is 1 key to facial beauty. The periocular region often displays marked asymmetry, particularly in the shape and position of the brow, eyelid margin, eyelid skin fold, and cheek and globe prominence. In Rhodes' study of facial symmetry,[4] the photos of digitally mirror-image faces were found to be more attractive than the unaltered asymmetric ones. Symmetry was found to correlate with perceived attractiveness.

The importance of symmetry to the facial surgeon cannot be overstated. All patients have a degree of facial asymmetry, however, many lack awareness of it. It is the surgeon's responsibility to photograph and document these asymmetries preoperatively, and to thoroughly discuss with the patient their impact on the surgical plan and projected outcome. Patients must understand that there will be some asymmetry postoperatively. These issues should be discussed preoperatively, and the patient must acknowledge the surgeon's concerns regarding asymmetry and the ability of surgery to address it.

The concept of averageness holds that the average facial features of a particular population form the ideal. This theory was evaluated by Langlois and Roggman,[5] comparing photos of individuals to the average computer-generated composite images of the group. Their results showed that the composites were rated as more attractive. Trujillo and coauthors[6] demonstrated that these average faces are recognized as human more readily and with less neural processing. Similarly, the Virtual Miss Germany project, performed at the University of Regensburg, morphed the faces of 22 Miss Germany finalists into 1 digital composite face. When compared with the face of the actual winner, the composite Virtual Miss Germany was selected as more attractive by all examiners.[7]

There are a number of equations and proposed ideal proportions suggested for the beautiful face. Swift and Remington[8] have proposed the mathematical ratio "phi" to describe many of these relationships in the face and body (**Fig. 7**). There are some anatomic features that, in deviating from the

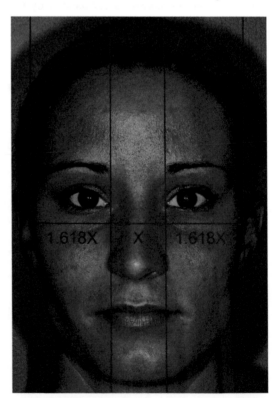

Fig. 7. Ideal facial proportions conforming to the ratio "Phi" 1.618. Ratio of intercanthal distance:sagittal width is Phi.

norm, tend to enhance beauty.[9] Their results suggest that female face attractiveness is greater when the face is symmetric, is close to the average, and has large eyes, prominent cheekbones, thick lips, thin eyebrows, and a small nose and chin.

The appearance of the skin surface is the first indicator of health and beauty when observing a face. Good skin tone and clarity can change the perception of an average face to an exceptional one. Skin should be uniform and smooth, without fine wrinkles or deeper rhytids, free of blemishes, with no dyschromias or abrupt changes in quality, texture, or contour. Averageness is a bonus here, and creating an even, smooth skin surface is a traditional role for cosmetics.

EYELID AESTHETICS

The upper eyelids display a gently curved lid margin, more acutely angled medially, with a peak height displaced toward the lateral limbus. Combined with the lower eyelid contour, this achieves a desirable almond shape of the palpebral fissure. Centrally, the upper eyelid margin falls just below the corneal limbus, with no superior scleral show.[10] The upper eyelid should be full, with neither fat pad protrusion, nor superior sulcus hollowing. The lashes should be long and thick, with a gentle outward curve.

Goldberg and Lew[11] have studied preoperative and postoperative measurements following blepharoplasty and repair of blepharoptosis, noting not only margin reflex distance (MRD) from a light reflex on the central cornea to the upper eyelid margin, but also the segment of skin exposed above the lashes in frontal view, which they defined as tarsal plate show (TPS) and the distance from the resting eyelid fold to the inferior brow, which they termed the brow fat span (BFS) (**Fig. 8**). They noted how ptosis repair shortens the TPS, and blepharoplasty increases TPS and decreases BFS. Further studies[12] categorized aging changes in the eyelid and reviewed the treatment of eyelid and orbital volume use with injectable hyaluronate fillers. Additional studies of the senior author (R.A. Goldberg, MD, personal communication, 2014) have used drawings with anomalies or asymmetries of the MRD, TPS, and BFS to assess the recognition of eyelid defects, suggesting that symmetry of TPS is more important than MRD symmetry in the perception of facial appearance. The weight of the upper lid tissues on the eyelid can be altered with frontalis tone lifting the brow. The position of the lid margin can be altered as much as 2 mm by altering the weight of these tissues with varied brow position.[13]

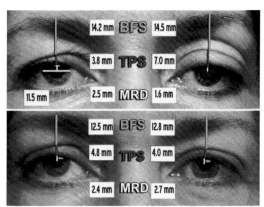

Fig. 8. Top, demonstration of measurement of BFS, TPS, and margin reflex distance (MRD1) on standardized photographs (corneal diameter set at 11.5 mm for scale). Bottom, in the same patient, following left ptosis surgery and bilateral asymmetric blepharoplasty, TPS symmetry has improved and BFS has shortened. (*From* Goldberg RA, Lew H. Cosmetic outcome of posterior approach ptosis surgery (an American Ophthalmologic Society thesis). Trans Am Ophthalmol Soc 2011;109:159; with permission.)

One can look at the classic measurements of lid crease height and contour, but it is ultimately the height and contour of the TPS and BFS that characterize the appearance of the open eyelid. Morley and colleagues[12] studied the TPS:BFS ratio, in relation to the use of fillers to add soft tissue volume to the superior sulcus and brow. The youthful eye has a long, full, straight TPS and BFS in a 1.0:1.5 ratio medially and a 1.0:3.0 ratio laterally (female patient) (**Fig. 9**). In the male patient, the lateral arch of the brow is less and the ratio more constant. Aging can change the ratios by increasing the TPS, as in blepharoptosis, or by decreasing it, as seen in brow ptosis and dermatochalasis. The eyelid crease tends to be slightly lower in men, and is often markedly lower or absent in Asian patients. A thorough discussion of patient expectations and desires pertaining to eyelid crease and skin fold configuration must be held preoperatively. This is especially true with the Asian blepharoplasty patient.

EYEBROW AESTHETICS

The brow is not only a feature that can convey youth and beauty, but also a common relay of emotion. Knoll[14] used simple line drawings to test observers' perceptions of emotion. Botulinum toxin treatment lessens the prominent glabellar furrows or frown lines that contribute to an aged or angry look. Increased or decreased tarsal plate show, along with depression of the lateral brow, was found to correlate with a perception of tiredness. A simulation

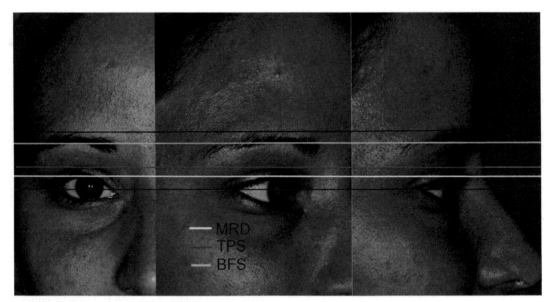

Fig. 9. Guide to eyelid, brow, and hairline position showing TPS:BFS ratio and hairline position.

of skin resection in blepharoplasty increased an observer's perception of tiredness.

As the tear trough frames the lower and lateral orbit, the eyebrow frames the superior orbit. Women begin to pluck and shape their brows at an early age in many cultures to project youth, beauty, or alertness. As a makeup artist, Westmore[15] lectured to plastic surgeons in the 1970s regarding his concepts of the ideal female brow position, as a gentle curve, with an apex above bony rim superior to the lateral corneal limbus and a medial edge aligned with the medial canthus and the lateral aspect of the nasal ala. The lateral brow would lie at the orbital rim where it intersects a line from the alar base through the lateral canthus (**Fig. 10**). The eyebrow tapers laterally, with appropriate vertical width of the brow cilia. There is a gradual transition from thick subbrow to thin upper eyelid skin. There are gender variations, with a generally thicker, and lower positioned tail of the eyebrow in men.

The aesthetically optimal location of the high point in the arc of the female brow has been a subject of much debate and numerous studies. Locations from the lateral limbus extending laterally to the lateral canthus are suggested,[15–18] with Pham[19] and colleagues placing the apex of the temporal brow curve at the temporal fusion line. Whitaker[16] felt the ideal male brow should be lower and straighter. He also placed peak of brow height in men at the junction of the middle third and lateral third of the brow.

Optimal perceived brow position and contour has changed over the decades and changes with the age of the individual grading beauty. A high arched, thinly plucked brow with a central apex was favored

from the 1930 through 1970's.[20–22] Ellenbogen[17] promoted a high brow position with the medial head 1 cm above the bony rim. Fashion magazines now show thicker low-set brows with a full subbrow fat pad.[23,24] In Feser's 2007 study,[25] younger individuals tended to favor this modern formulation of beauty, while those over age 50 preferred the older aesthetic.

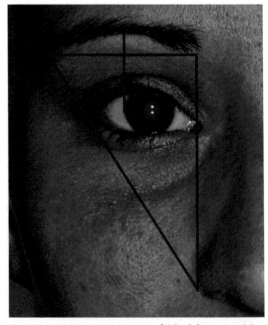

Fig. 10. Westmore's concept of ideal brow position showing high point of arch at lateral limbus and position of head and tail of brow.

AGING CHANGES

Skin changes, bony and soft tissue changes, and soft tissue descent all contribute to the appearance of facial aging. Brow ptosis and volume loss, dermatochalasis, blepharoptosis, lacrimal gland prolapse, and fat prolapse all occur with age. Pottier[26] noted the loss of elastin and collagen in the eyelid skin, with a preservation of the orbicularis muscle leading to folds, rhytids, and an indistinct eyelid crease. The alternate aged upper eyelid appearance related to involutional blepharoptosis results in an elevated eyelid crease with retracted preaponeurotic fat giving the aged appearance of a hollow orbit. The degree to which involutional changes of the levator aponeurosis affects the upper lid sulcus is vital to determine in the aging eyelid to plan appropriate treatment. Korn and colleagues[27] noted the increase in medial fat and decrease in central upper eyelid fat with age, beginning in the fourth decade and most significant from the seventh decade onward. The medial orbital fat resembles the posterior orbital fat, with numerous stem cells that are relatively preserved. The central fat pad resembles body fat more and is relatively less conserved in most patients with age.

The traditional approach to upper blepharoplasty entails a resection of presumably redundant skin, muscle, and fat from the upper eyelid. Overly aggressive resection, especially centrally, may result in a hollow central superior sulcus.[2,12] Improved understanding of periorbital physiology from aging has led to modified blepharoplasty techniques. Periorbital volume restoration and augmentation, instead of reduction, are increasingly popular among cosmetic surgeons using fat conservation and repositioning with orbicularis oculi muscle preservation in upper blepharoplasty.[23,26–29]

There are other possible causes for bulging and prolapse of tissue in the lateral eyelid, including a prolapsed lacrimal gland that is severe in approximately 10% of upper blepharoplasty patients.[30] This can be identified as a mobile mass in the lateral upper lid that prolapses further with globe pressure. The lacrimal gland should not be resected, but it can be reposited in the 5% to 10% of patients in whom it is warranted. Resection of the lacrimal gland should be avoided, as it can interfere with tear production.

A great deal of emphasis has been placed in recent years on the loss or redistribution of facial fat with age. Using photographic documentation over a period of decades, Lambros[31] demonstrated a slight descent of the eyebrows, hollowing of the temples, periorbital hollowing, and lateral shift of the peak of the upper eyelid margin with blepharoptosis and/or dermatochalasis. The lateral canthus shifts medially, with the medial canthus relatively fixed, shortening the horizontal palpebral fissure. Rohrich and Pessa[32] made complementary anatomic observations on the loss of volume in facial fat compartments causing collapse and descent in aging.

Bony changes with aging appear to contribute to facial aging changes. Enlargement of the skull and frontal sinuses may increase the prominence of the supraorbital bar.[33,34] An increase in the size of the orbital aperture, as described by Pessa,[35] occurs along with a widening superomedially and inferolaterally. This opening of the orbit will contribute to prominence of the tear trough inferiorly and the medial fat pad superiorly. Repositioning of the medial fat pad in the upper lid and glabella has been described to address this superomedial orbital change.[30,36] The lack of bony support may contribute to the volume loss under the brow and descent of the brow tissues.[37] Although surgical techniques to directly address these changes exist, surgeons are still working through finding the optimal paradigms to address aesthetic changes induced by aging of the facial skeleton.

The temporal brow descends with age,[2,16,31,38] with significant temporal volume loss and a lack of frontalis muscle function to elevate the lateral brow. Many aging patients use tonic frontalis muscle tone to maintain a brow position adequate for vision[39] and brow position may paradoxically raise with age.[39,40] In many patients, the reduction in dermatochalasis overhanging the upper lid margin attained by tonic frontalis tone is important functionally and cosmetically. Overzealous treatment of forehead rhytids with botulinum toxin will result in a symptomatic and bothersome increase in dermatochalasis. Likewise, upper blepharoplasty in such a patient as a stand-alone procedure may result in the relaxation of frontalis tone and a significant and newly apparent brow ptosis.

SUMMARY

There are several general characteristics and specific anatomic relationships that affect one's perception of attractiveness in the periocular region. Aging occurs in somewhat predictable patterns. Changes in the skin, fat compartments and other soft tissues, and facial skeleton all contribute to the appearance of an aging face. An understanding of the anatomy aging changes and one's perception of those changes can lead to more appropriate therapy. Although some of these aging factors are amenable to medical or surgical alteration, others are not. An understanding of what is considered beautiful can shape one's approach to the evaluation and management of patients seeking facial rejuvenation.

REFERENCES

1. Lam VB, Czyz CN, Wulc AE. The brow-lid continuum: an anatomic perspective. Clin Plast Surg 2013;40:1–19.
2. Hartstein ME, Kikkawa D. How to avoid blepharoplasty complications. Oral Maxillofac Surg Clin North Am 2009;21:31–41.
3. Buchanan AG, Holds JB. The beautiful eye: perception of beauty in the periocular area. Chapter 3. In: Paul MD, Hovsepian RV, Rotunda AM, editors. Master techniques in blepharoplasty and periorbital rejuvenation. Springer Science + Business Media; 2011. p. 25–9.
4. Rhodes G, Profitt F, Grady JM, et al. Facial symmetry and the perception of beauty. Psychon Bull Rev 1998;5:659–69.
5. Langlois JH, Roggman LA. Attractive faces are only average. Psychol Sci 1990;1:115–21.
6. Trujillo LT, Jankowitsch JM, Langlois JH. Beauty is in the ease of the beholding: a neurophysiological test of the averageness theory of facial attractiveness. Cogn Affect Behav Neurosci 2014;14(3):1061–76.
7. Braun C, Gruendl M, Marberger C, et al. 2001. Available at: http://www.uni-Beautycheck-rsachen.und.Folgen.von.Attraktivitaet.regensburg.de/Fakultaeten/phil_Fak_II/Psychologie/Psy_II/beautycheck/english/bericht/bericht.htm.
8. Swift A, Remington K. BeautiPHIcation: a global approach to facial beauty. Clin Plast Surg 2011;38(3):347–77.
9. Baudouin JY, Tiberghian G. Symmetry, averageness, and feature size in facial attractiveness of women. Acta Psychol (Amst) 2004;117(3):313–32.
10. Shorr N, Enzer YR. Considerations in aesthetic eyelid surgery. J Dermatol Surg Oncol 1992;18(12):1081–95.
11. Goldberg RA, Lew H. Cosmetic outcome of posterior approach ptosis surgery (an American Ophthalmological Society thesis). Trans Am Ophthalmol Soc 2011;109:157–67.
12. Morley AM, Taban M, Malhotra R, et al. Use of hyaluronic acid gel for upper eyelid filling and contouring. Ophthal Plast Reconstr Surg 2009;25:440–4.
13. Karacalar A. Compensatory brow asymmetry: anatomic study and clinical experience. Aesthetic Plast Surg 2005;29(2):119–23.
14. Knoll B, Attkiss KJ, Persing JA. The influence of forehead, brow, and periorbital aesthetics on perceived expression in the youthful face. Plast Reconstr Surg 2008;121:1793.
15. Westmore M. Facial cosmetics in conjunction with surgery. Presented at Aesthetic Plastic Surgical Society Meeting. Vancouver, Canada, May 7, 1974.
16. Whitaker LA, Morales L Jr, Farkas LG. Aesthetic surgery of the supraorbital ridge and forehead structures. Plast Reconstr Surg 1986;78(1):23–32.
17. Ellenbogen R. Transcoronal eyebrow lift with concomitant upper blepharoplasty. Plast Reconstr Surg 1983;71(4):490–9.
18. Cook TA. The versatile midforehead browlift. Arch Otolaryngol Head Neck Surg 1989;115(2):163–8.
19. Pham S, Wilhelmi B, Mowlavi A. Eyebrow peak position redefined. Aesthet Surg J 2010;30(3):297–300.
20. Oestreicher JH, Hurwitz JJ. The position of the eyebrow. Ophthalmic Surg 1990;21(4):245–9.
21. Romm S. The changing face of beauty. Aesthetic Plast Surg 1989;13(2):91–8.
22. Volpe CR, Ramirez OM. The beautiful eye. Facial Plast Surg Clin North Am 2005;13(4):493–504.
23. Fagien S. Advanced rejuvenative upper blepharoplasty: enhancing aesthetics of the upper periorbita. Plast Reconstr Surg 2002;110(1):278–91 [discussion: 292].
24. Rohrich RJ. Current concepts in aesthetic upper blepharoplasty. Plast Reconstr Surg 2004;113(3):32e–42e.
25. Feser DK. Attractiveness of eyebrow position and shape in females depends on the age of the beholder. Aesthetic Plast Surg 2007;31(2):154–60.
26. Pottier F, El-Shazly NZ, El-Shazly AE. Aging of orbicularis oculi: anatomophysiologic consideration in upper blepharoplasty. Arch Facial Plast Surg 2008;10(5):346–9.
27. Korn BS, Kikkawa DO, Hicok KC. Identification and characterization of adult stem cells from human orbital adipose tissue. Ophthal Plast Reconstr Surg 2009;25:27–32.
28. Oh SR, Chokthaweesak W, Annunziata CC, et al. Analysis of eyelid fat pad changes with aging. Ophthal Plast Reconstr Surg 2011;27:348–51.
29. Massry GG. Nasal fat preservation in upper eyelid blepharoplasty. Ophthal Plast Reconstr Surg 2011;27(5):352–5.
30. Massry GG. Prevalence of lacrimal gland prolapse in the functional blepharoplasty population. Ophthal Plast Reconstr Surg 2011;27(6):410–3.
31. Lambros V. Observations on periorbital and midface aging. Plast Reconstr Surg 2007;120(5):1367–76 [discussion: 1377].
32. Rohrich RJ, Pessa JE. The fat compartments of the face: anatomy and clinical implications for cosmetic surgery. Plast Reconstr Surg 2007;119(7):2219–27 [discussion: 2228–31].
33. Bartlett SP, Grossman R, Whitaker LA. Age-related changes of the craniofacial skeleton: an anthropometric and histologic analysis. Plast Reconstr Surg 1992;90(4):592–600.
34. Israel H. The dichotomous pattern of craniofacial expansion during aging. Am J Phys Anthropol 1977;47(1):47–51.
35. Pessa JE, Chen Y. Curve analysis of the aging orbital aperture. Plast Reconstr Surg 2002;109(2):751–5 [discussion: 756–60].
36. Yoo DB, Peng GL, Massry GG. Effacing the orbitoglabellar groove with transposed upper eyelid fat. Ophthal Plast Reconstr Surg 2013;29(3):220–4.

37. Kahn DM, Shaw RB. Overview of current thoughts on facial volume and aging. Facial Plast Surg 2010;26(5):350–5.

38. Knize DM. An anatomically based study of the mechanism of eyebrow ptosis. Plast Reconstr Surg 1996;97(7):1321–33.

39. Matros E, Garcia JA, Yaremchuk MJ. Changes in eyebrow position and shape with aging. Plast Reconstr Surg 2009;124(4):1296–301.

40. van den Bosch WA, Leenders I, Mulder P. Topographic anatomy of the eyelids, and the effects of sex and age. Br J Ophthalmol 1999;83(3):347–52.

Midface Anatomy, Aging, and Aesthetic Analysis

Andre Yuan Levesque, MD[a], Jorge I. de la Torre, MD[b],*

KEYWORDS

- Midface anatomy • Facial aging • Aesthetic analysis • Malar fat pad • Sub–orbicularis oculi fat

KEY POINTS

- The midface is the region between the upper and lower thirds of the face. Within the midface there is an anterior portion referred to as the midcheek and the posterior portion referred to as the lateral cheek.
- The changes with aging tend to affect the midcheek structures with laxity of the soft tissue supporting ligaments (orbitomalar, zygomatic, and masseteric), bony atrophy, decreases in skin thickness elasticity, and subcutaneous fat resorption.
- Goals in midface rejuvenation are to produce midcheek fullness and smooth transition into adjacent areas of the lower lid and lower face.

DEFINITION OF THE AREA

The midface is commonly used to describe the central third of the face because it is commonly divided into the upper, middle, and lower face. The upper border of the midface extends from the superior helix along the upper zygomatic arch to the lateral canthus and then along the lower lid to the nose. The lower border extends from the lower tragus to the oral commissure and along the nasolabial fold to the nose (**Fig. 1**).[1,2] The midface can further be divided by a line from the lateral canthus to the commissure. Anterior to the line is the midcheek and posterior is the lateral cheek.

The midcheek and can further be divided into lid-cheek, malar, and nasolabial components (**Fig. 2**). The palpebral malar crease separates the lower lid and malar fat divisions. The nasojugal crease separates the lower lid and nasolabial divisions. The midcheek furrow separates the malar and nasolabial divisions.[2]

With aging, the midcheek divisions become apparent with development of a nasojugal fold medially, palpebral malar groove superolaterally, and a midcheek furrow inferolaterally in the shape of a Y in between the 3 components of the midcheek (**Fig. 3**).[2,3] The youthful midcheek typically blends into the lower lid, nose, nasolabial, and lateral facial regions without demarcation and has uniform fullness and volume.[1,2]

With further anatomic study the superficial fat of the cheek itself has been shown to have 3 separate fat compartments: the medial, middle, and lateral temporal compartments, which all have separate septae.[4] In addition, the sub–orbicularis oculi fat (SOOF) located in the lid-cheek division has also been shown to have 2 separate fat compartments. The medial component of the SOOF extends from the medial limbus to the lateral canthus along the orbital rim and the lateral component extends from the medial fat pad to the temporal fat pad.[5]

Disclosure: None of the authors have any pertinent financial disclosures related to the content of this article.
[a] Division of Plastic Surgery, University of Alabama at Birmingham, 1158 Faculty Office Tower, 510 20th Street South, Birmingham, AL 35210, USA; [b] Division of Plastic Surgery, Birmingham VA Medical Center, University of Alabama at Birmingham, 1102 Faculty Office Tower, 510 20th Street South, Birmingham, AL 35210, USA
* Corresponding author.
E-mail address: jdlt@uab.edu

facialplastic.theclinics.com

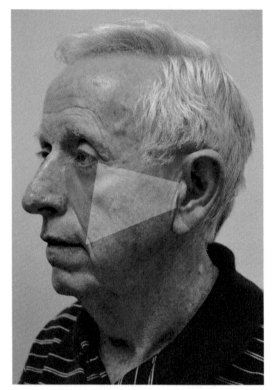

Fig. 1. The superior border of the midface lies along a line from the root of the helix to the lateral canthus to medial canthus along the side of the nose. The inferior border can be thought of as a line from the inferior border of the tragus to the lateral commissure along the nasolabial fold to the nose. The midcheek (*blue*) lies anterior to a line from the lateral canthus to commissure and posterior lies the lateral cheek (*green*).

INTERNAL ORGANIZATION/LAYERS OF THE AREA

The layers in the midface are similar to those in the upper and lower face with skin, subcutaneous fat, a musculoaponeurotic layer, loose areolar layer, and periosteum/bone (**Figs. 4 and 5**).[2]

The bony framework consists of the zygoma and the maxillary bones with a small component of the lacrimal bone.[6] Important attachments to the bony framework are the mimetic muscles, the zygomaticus major and minor, and the zygomatic ligament arising between and around the zygomaticus major and minor and minor muscles. There is limited bone available for attachment of soft tissue because the oral cavity mucosal reflexion occupies a large portion of the anterior maxilla. In addition, the prezygomatic space with the orbito-malar ligament superior and zygomatic ligaments inferiorly also limits direct soft tissue attachment to the zygomatic bone.[2] This arrangement allows gliding of the soft tissues over the spaces and

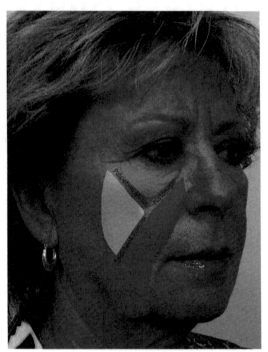

Fig. 2. The portions of the midcheek divided into lid-cheek (*blue*), nasolabial (*red*) extending into the jowl, and malar (*green*) separated by the palpebral malar crease, nasojugal crease, and midcheek furrow.

allows the separate functions of eye closure, smiling, and chewing.

In the midcheek region immediate superficial to the maxilla and zygoma lies the deep fat compartment, with preperiosteal fat and the buccal fat pad. This fat lies deep to the zygomaticus muscles and

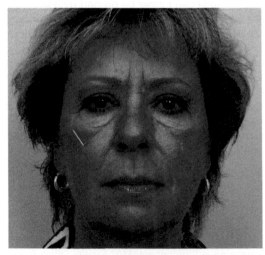

Fig. 3. Note superomedial nasojugal folds (*blue*), superolateral palpebral malar groove (*green*), infero-lateral midcheek furrow (*red*), which form the shape of a Y on anterior view.

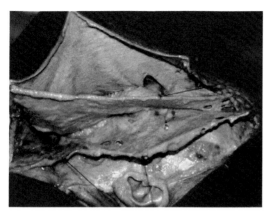

Fig. 4. Cadaver dissection showing separation of skin, subcutaneous fat, superficial musculoaponeurotic system (SMAS), and deeper structures.

levator labii superioris, and within the fat pad are terminal branches of the zygomatic and buccal nerves that pass more superficially to innervate their muscle targets in the musculoaponeurotic layer.[7] This layer allows gliding of the mimetic muscles (zygomaticus major and minor, levator labii superioris) with facial expressions. The zygomatic nerve innervates the zygomatic muscles on their deep surface but more medially innervates the levator superioris on its superficial surface.

The superficial musculoaponeurotic system (SMAS), often credited to Mitz and Peyronie,[8] is a distinct layer in the face that is more developed

in the lateral cheek region and becomes less distinct into the anterior face or midcheek region. Laterally the SMAS is more distinct separate from the parotid fascia and is continuous with the platysma inferiorly and the temporoparietal fascia superiorly.[8] The SMAS also separates fat into a superficial fat compartment that contains septae and a deeper fat compartment without septae. In the midcheek region this is analogous to the SMAS/mimetic muscle layer separating the malar fat pad from the buccal fat pad. The exact relationship of the SMAS with the parotid fascia and mimetic muscles is not clearly shown in all studies, but most studies agree that the SMAS is most distinct in the parotid region and becomes thin and less substantial moving anterior into the midcheek region.[8–11]

The subcutaneous layer in the midface includes the malar fat pad, which can be further subdivided into 3 separate compartments (medial, middle, and lateral), and each can age differently.[4] Superior and deep to the malar fat pad is the SOOF,[12] which occupies the prezygomatic space between the orbitomalar ligament and zygomatic ligament with the roof of the space being the orbicularis oculi muscle.[1,2,5] The SOOF is separate and distinct from the malar fat and adherent to the deep surface of the orbicular oculi muscle, whereas the malar fat pad is superficial to the SMAS.

SURROUNDING AREAS

The lower lid has distinct function and anatomy and can be treated in isolation or with the midface. The orbital malar ligament serves as the dividing layer with the midcheek and the lower lid structures above. In the lower lid, the layers can be separated into 3 lamellae. The anterior lamella consists of the skin and orbicularis oculi muscle, the middle lamella is the orbital septum and fat. The posterior lamella contains the tarsus, conjunctiva, and lower lid retractors.[13] The lower lid orbital fat has 3 compartments with the medial, central, and temporal fat pads (**Fig. 6**). The inferior oblique

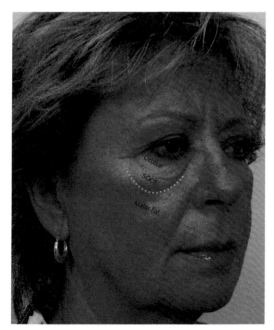

Fig. 5. Relationship of the orbital fat, orbitomalar ligament (*blue*), SOOF, zygomatic ligament (*green*), and malar fat with surface bulges and creases.

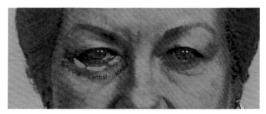

Fig. 6. The lower lid orbital fat is separated into 3 compartments: medial, central, and temporal. The inferior oblique muscle separates the medial and central compartments and can be damaged inadvertently.

muscle separates the medial and central fat pads and can inadvertently be damaged during surgery.[14]

Development of a jowl is a result of descent of cheek soft tissues from attenuation of the masseteric ligaments.[15] The described lower premasseteric space can be useful in describing the changes involved in developing a jowl. The roof of the space is the platysma and SMAS and the inferior border is a membranous connection from the SMAS layer to the mandible that anteriorly connects to the mandibular ligament. With aging, the development of laxity in SMAS, platysma, inferior border of the space, and lower masseteric ligaments allows the roof to slide and the superficial fat to descend beneath the level of the mandible, producing the jowl (**Fig. 7**).[16]

LIGAMENTS

The idea of retaining ligaments of the face or connection from bone or fascia to the dermis was proposed and demonstrated by Furnas.[17] It was further developed by Mendelson,[1] Rohrich and Pessa,[4,18] and others. The important ligaments within the midface are the zygomatic ligaments, orbitomalar ligament, and masseteric ligaments. The confluence of the 3 cheek fat compartments has commonly been described as the zygomatic ligament. In addition, the confluence of the medial and middle cheek compartments has been described as the masseteric ligaments (**Figs. 8 and 9**).[4]

Between the ligaments there is minimal attachment of the soft tissue to the underlying skeleton allowing movement and facial expression. This minimal attachment also provides an opportunity for repositioning of tissue through surgical manipulation and a safe, expeditious plane of dissection. In

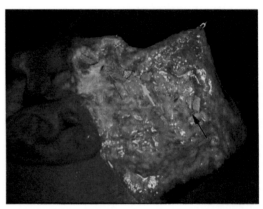

Fig. 8. Cadaver dissection showing the zygomatic ligaments (*red arrow*), the masseteric ligaments (*green arrow*), and the mandibular ligament (*black arrow*) at the anterior border of the masseter deep to the SMAS.

sub-SMAS dissection there are safe planes of dissection overlying the masseter, divided into the upper, middle, and lower premasseteric spaces, to reach the anterior space as described by Mendelson and colleagues[16] and Mendelson and Wong.[19]

BLOOD SUPPLY

The blood supply to the midface arises from the external carotid artery and its branches via the facial artery and transverse facial arteries. The maxillary artery supplies the muscles and deeper

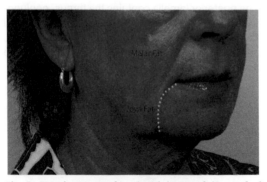

Fig. 7. Development of jowl with laxity of the roof of the premasseteric space SMAS/platysma and masseteric ligaments (*red stars*) with persistent fixation of the mandibular ligament (*black star*). The labiomandibular fold is outlined in green.

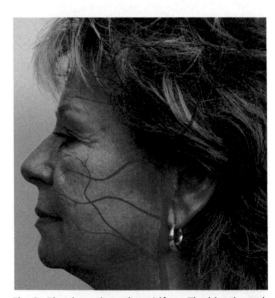

Fig. 9. Blood supply to the midface. The blood supply derives from the external carotid largely by way of the facial, maxillary, and transverse facial arteries and veins.

structures of the face via the buccal and infra-orbital arteries. Venous drainage accompanies the arteries as separately named veins as well as vena comitans, and ultimately draining into the internal jugular system.[6]

The anterior portion of the midface is supplied via musculocutaneous perforators through the facial mimetic muscles arising from the facial artery system through the facial mimetic muscles. The lateral portion of the midface is typically provided via fasciocutaneous perforators from the transverse facial artery.[20,21]

LYMPHATICS

The lymphatics of the midface drain to the submental and submandibular nodes but form a rich plexus of lymphatics more dense than that of the scalp. The lymphatics begin in the subcutaneous space as lymph capillaries and drain into precollecting lymph vessels, collecting lymphatics, and then the first-tier lymph nodes. The first-tier lymph nodes are generally situated deep along the deep veins of the face and neck.[22,23]

The facial lymph nodes are the infraorbital, buccinator, and maxillary nodes, which most commonly drain to the submandibular nodes (**Fig. 10**). Disruption of the lymphatic system can

lead to prolonged swelling either from direct transection or from pressure on the lymphatic system from filler materials.[24,25] Swelling can be most visible superior to the orbital malar ligament because the ligament is largely impermeable and serves as a barrier for fluid, blood, or lymph to accumulate and form festoons, malar mounds, malar edema, and periorbital ecchymosis.[23]

INNERVATION

The anatomy of the facial nerve is described in many publications but, specific to midface anatomy, the depth and location of the terminal sections of the zygomatic and buccal branches are important to understand to avoid injury. The zygomatic and buccal branches emerge from the parotid beneath the deep investing parotid fascia and travel more superficially as the nerve progresses more anteriorly.[26] The branches then lie immediately deep to the SMAS layer until innervating their muscle targets on the deep surface (zygomaticus major and minor, orbicularis oculi) and then through the SMAS layer to innervate the levator labii superioris (**Fig. 11**). Dissection

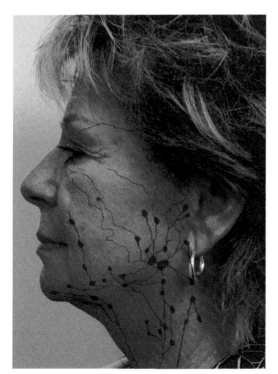

Fig. 10. Lymphatic system within the midface. Typically following the venous system, the important lymph nodes are the infraorbital, buccinator, and maxillary nodes, which drain to the submandibular nodes.

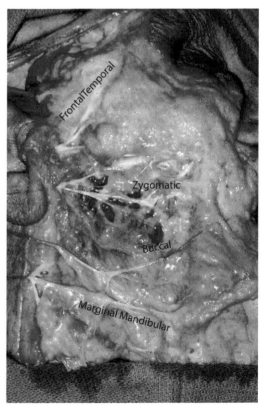

Fig. 11. The course of the extratemporal facial nerve in the face. The zygomatic and buccal branches are the important branches for midface rejuvenation.

within the subcutaneous space should be safe at all times except when overlying the levator muscles, but care must be taken with sub-SMAS dissection to avoid the zygomatic and buccal branches that traverse the sub-SMAS space. Similarly, a deeper plane of dissection also protects the facial nerve branches, as in a subperiosteal approach to the midface. In the midface in particular there are significant cross-innervations between zygomatic and buccal nerves, with about 50% cross-innervations, and damage to one branch is likely to result in no functional consequence.[27]

Sensation to the midface skin is provided mainly by branches of the infraorbital and zygomaticofacial nerves. In addition, there are minor contributions from the zygomaticotemporal nerve, infratrochlear nerve, auricular temporal nerve, and buccal nerve.[6]

SURGICAL ANATOMIC CONSIDERATIONS

The critical structure of the midface with respect to midface rejuvenation is the malar fat pad. The malar fat pad is located between the SMAS and the skin and is firmly attached to the skin.[28] The youthful position of the malar fat pad is characterized by positioning over the zygomatic arch with the superior portion covering the orbital portion of the orbicularis oculi muscle and inferior portion at the nasolabial fold with no bulging anterior to the fold.[29] With appropriate repositioning of the malar fat pad in a superior vector, the lower lid vertical distance is decreased and hollowness is eliminated in the infraorbital region.

Approaching the midface from a hairline incision can be accomplished in a subcutaneous plane and sub-SMAS plane. The subcutaneous plane is inherently safe because the branches of the facial nerve are protected by the SMAS. In a sub-SMAS plane, if the prezygomatic space is respected and properly developed, the zygomatic branch and buccal branches should be protected by the walls of the space.[19] Vascularity to the overlying skin should be robust in the same fashion as a facelift flap survives with extensive undermining.[20,21] The malar fat pad can then be resuspended in a vertical direction by the subcutaneous exposure and fixed to the temporal fascia.[28]

The midface can also be approached from periorbital approaches and even percutaneously, and all approaches are safe when the appropriate layers of dissection are respected either superficial to SMAS, subperiosteal, or in the prezygomatic spaces. A myriad of techniques for midface correction have been proposed and most can be effective and safe, and readers should refer to the literature for the details of the individual procedures.[28,30–33]

IMAGING

Computed tomography scan or plain radiographs typically have little utility in preoperative planning for rejuvenation of the midface; however, excellent standard reproducible photographs should be the goal. Close-up views of the face should be obtained with anterior, oblique, lateral, upward gaze, closed eyes, and worms-eye views. Full-face photographs should also be obtained in anterior, oblique, and lateral views. We also like to take an animation photograph with the patient smiling for midface anaylsis.[34,35]

SUMMARY

Attention to the changes within the midface is critical to achieve a harmonious facial rejuvenation. Global changes in all layers of the midface occur to produce signs of aging. The bony framework undergoes resorption with time, especially in edentulous patients.[36–42] The orbitomalar, zygomatic, and masseteric ligaments all develop laxity and allow descent of the attached soft tissues. There is also typically some loss in fat and skin thickness. Surgical correction of the midface should be directed at all layers and particular care given to blending changes into the adjacent regions of the lower lid and lower face. The anatomy, although complex because of the small spaces involved, is well described and with appropriate study surgical correction of the midface can be safe and effective.

REFERENCES

1. Mendelson BC, Muzaffar AR, Adams WP Jr. Surgical anatomy of the midcheek and malar mounds. Plast Reconstr Surg 2002;110(3):885–96.
2. Mendelson BC, Jacobson SR. Surgical anatomy of the midcheek: facial layers, spaces, and the midcheek segments. Clin Plast Surg 2008;35(3): 395–404.
3. Tan KS, Oh SR, Priel A, et al. Surgical anatomy of the forehead, eyelids, and midface for the aesthetic surgeon. In: Massry GG, Murphy MR, Azizzadeh B, editors. Master techniques in blepharoplasty and periorbital rejuvenation. New York: Springer; 2011. p. 11–24.
4. Rohrich RJ, Pessa JE. The fat compartments of the face: anatomy and clinical implications for cosmetic surgery. Plast Reconstr Surg 2007;119(7):2219–27.
5. Rohrich RJ, Arbique GM, Wong C, et al. The anatomy of suborbicularis fat: implications for periorbital rejuvenation. Plast Reconstr Surg 2009;124:946–51.
6. Netter FH. Atlas of human anatomy. 6th edition. Philadelphia: Saunders; 2014.

7. Gassner HG, Rafii A, Young A, et al. Surgical anatomy of the face implications for modern face-lift techniques. Arch Facial Plast Surg 2008; 10(1):9–19.

8. Mitz V, Peyronie M. The superficial musculo-aponeurotic system (SMAS) in the parotid and cheek area. Plast Reconstr Surg 1976;58(1):80–8.

9. Gardetto A, Dabernig J, Rainer C, et al. Does a superficial musculoaponeurotic system exist in the face and neck? An anatomical study by the tissue plastination technique. Plast Reconstr Surg 2003; 111(2):664–72.

10. Gosain AK, Yousif NJ, Madiedo G, et al. Surgical anatomy of the SMAS: a reinvestigation. Plast Reconstr Surg 1993;92(7):1254–63.

11. Thaller SR, Kim S, Patterson H, et al. The submuscular aponeurotic system (SMAS): a histologic and comparative anatomy evaluation. Plast Reconstr Surg 1990;86(4):690–6.

12. Aiache AE, Ramirez OH. The suborbicularis oculi fat pads: an anatomic and clinical study. Plast Reconstr Surg 1995;95(1):37–42.

13. Kakizaki H, Malhotra R, Madge SN, et al. Lower eyelid anatomy: an update. Ann Plast Surg 2009; 63:344–51.

14. Mowlavi A, Neumeister MW, Wilhelmi BJ. Lower blepharoplasty using bony anatomical landmarks to identify and avoid injury to the inferior oblique muscle. Plast Reconstr Surg 2002;110:1318–22.

15. Stuzin JM, Baker TJ, Gordon HL. The relationship of the superficial and deep facial fascias: relevance to rhytidectomy and aging. Plast Reconstr Surg 1992; 89:441.

16. Mendelson BC, Freeman ME, Wu W, et al. Surgical anatomy of the lower face: the premasseter space, the jowl, and the labiomandibular fold. Aesthet Plast Surg 2008;32:185–95.

17. Furnas DW. The retaining ligaments of the cheek. Plast Reconstr Surg 1989;83:11–6.

18. Rohrich RJ, Pessa JE. The retaining system of the face: histologic evaluation of the septal boundaries of the subcutaneous fat compartments. Plast Reconstr Surg 2008;121(5):1804–9.

19. Mendelson BC, Wong CH. Surgical anatomy of the middle premasseter space and its application in sub-SMAS face lift surgery. Plast Reconstr Surg 2013;132:57–64.

20. Schaverien MV, Pessa JE, Saint-Cyr M, et al. The arterial and venous anatomies of the lateral face lift flap and the SMAS. Plast Reconstr Surg 2009; 123(5):1581–7.

21. Whetzel TP, Mathes SJ. The arterial supply of the face lift flap. Plast Reconstr Surg 1997;100:480–6.

22. Pan WR, Suami H, Taylor IG. Lymphatic drainage of the superficial tissues of the head and neck: anatomical study and clinical implications. Plast Reconstr Surg 2008;121:1614–24.

23. Pan WR, Le Roux CM, Briggs CA. Variations in the lymphatic drainage pattern of the head and neck: further anatomic studies and clinical implications. Plast Reconstr Surg 2011;127:611–20.

24. Funt DK. Avoiding malar edema during midface/cheek augmentation with dermal fillers. J Clin Aesthet Dermatol 2011;4(12):32–6.

25. Pessa JE, Garza JR. The malar septum: the anatomic basis of malar mounds and malar edema. Aesthet Surg J 1997;17(1):11–7.

26. Davis RA, Anson B, Jbudinger JM, et al. Surgical anatomy of the facial nerve and parotid gland based upon a study of 350 cervicofacial halves. Surg Gynecol Obstet 1956;102:385.

27. Gosain AK. Surgical anatomy of the facial nerve. Clin Plast Surg 1995;22(2):241–51.

28. De Cordier B, de la Torre J, Al-Hakeem M, et al. Rejuvenation of the midface by elevating the malar fat pad: review of technique, cases, and complications. Plast Reconstr Surg 2002;110: 1526–36.

29. Yousif N, Mendelson B. Anatomy of the midface. Clin Plast Surg 1995;22:227.

30. De la Torre JI, Martin SA, Vásconez LO. Suture suspension of the malar fat pad. Aesthet Surg J 2002; 22:446–50.

31. Verpaele A, Tonnard P, Gaia S, et al. The third suture in MACS-lifting: making midface-lifting simple and safe. J Plast Reconstr Aesthet Surg 2007;60: 1287–95.

32. Saltz R, Ohana B. Thirteen years of experience with the endoscopic midface lift. Aesthet Surg J 2012;32: 927–36.

33. Hamra ST. Arcus marginalis release and orbital fat preservation in midface rejuvenation. Plast Reconstr Surg 1995;96:354–62.

34. Henderson JL, Larrabee WF, Krieger BD. Photographic standards for facial plastic surgery. Arch Facial Plast Surg 2005;7:331–3.

35. DiBernardo BE, Adams RL, Krause J, et al. Photographic standards in plastic surgery. Plast Reconstr Surg 1998;102:559–68.

36. Kahn DM, Shaw RB Jr. Aging of the bony orbit: a three-dimensional computed tomographic study. Aesthet Surg J 2008;28:258–64.

37. Pessa JE, Chen Y. Curve analysis of the aging orbital aperture. Plast Reconstr Surg 2002;109:751–5.

38. Pessa JE. An algorithm of facial aging: verification of Lambros's theory by three-dimensional stereolithography, with reference to the pathogenesis of midfacial aging, scleral show, and the lateral suborbital trough deformity. Plast Reconstr Surg 2000;106: 479–88.

39. Shaw RB Jr, Kahn DM. Aging of the midface bony elements: a three-dimensional computed tomographic study. Plast Reconstr Surg 2007;119: 675–81.

40. Mendelson BC, Hartley W, Scott M, et al. Age-related changes of the orbit and midcheek and the implications for facial rejuvenation. Aesthet Plast Surg 2007;31:419–23.

41. Pessa JE, Zadoo VP, Yuan C, et al. Concertina effect and facial aging: nonlinear aspects of youthfulness and skeletal remodeling, and why, perhaps, infants have jowls. Plast Reconstr Surg 1999;103:635–44.

42. Pessa JE, Zadoo VP, Mutimer KL, et al. Relative maxillary retrusion as a natural consequence of aging: combining skeletal and soft tissue changes into an integrated model of midfacial aging. Plast Reconstr Surg 1998;102:205–12.

Minimally Invasive Surgical Adjuncts to Upper Blepharoplasty

César A. Briceño, MD[a], Sandy X. Zhang-Nunes, MD[b],
Guy G. Massry, MD[c],*

KEYWORDS

- Eyebrow anatomy • Eyelid anatomy • Browpexy • Upper eyelid blepharoplasty
- Upper eyelid fat preservation • Orbitoglabellar groove • Lacrimal gland prolapse
- Brassiere brow fat suspension

KEY POINTS

- Contemporary blepharoplasty surgery has undergone a paradigm shift which focuses on techniques that preserve volume.
- A browpexy is a minimally invasive, nonformal, temporal brow stabilization or conservative lift that can be performed in an external or internal fashion.
- The nasal fat pad of the upper eyelid is relatively stem cell–rich and tends to become clinically more prominent with age. This fat can be preserved and redistributed within and outside the eyelid/orbit during blepharoplasty.
- Lacrimal gland prolapse is a normal involutional change that can lead to temporal eyelid fullness. The gland be safely repositioned to its native location during blepharoplasty surgery.
- The brow fat pad can be elevated and supported during blepharoplasty surgery to potentially improve the eyebrow-eyelid transition and contour.

Video of (1) External Browpexy Procedure, (2) Nasal Fat Preservation, (3) Nasal Fat Preservation: Orbitoglabellar Groove, (4) Lacrimal Gland Repositioning, and (5) Brassiere Suture Fixation of Brow Fat Pad accompanyies this article at http://www.facialplastic.theclinics.com/

INTRODUCTION

Upper blepharoplasty is one of the most common facial aesthetic and functional procedures performed in the world today.[1] It is one of the oldest described treatments of the aging face;[2] initially elaborated on in ancient times by Albucasis in Spain,[3] and Ali Ibn Isa in Baghdad.[4] In these early reports, upper eyelid skin was grossly removed with cautery or pressure necrosis. Upper eyelid surgery was then largely forgotten until reemerging in the eighteenth and nineteenth centuries.[5] The procedure has evolved significantly into a technique that also addresses the orbicularis muscle and eyelid/orbital fat. In the 1950s, Costaneras[6] enhanced our understanding of contemporary

---

The authors have no financial disclosures.

[a] Department of Ophthalmology and Visual Sciences, Kellogg Eye Center, University of Michigan, 1000 Wall Street, Ann Arbor, MI 48105, USA; [b] Department of Ophthalmology, USC Eye Institute, University of Southern California, Keck School of Medicine, 1450 San Pablo Street, 4th floor, Los Angeles, CA 90033, USA; [c] Ophthalmic Plastic and Reconstructive Surgery, University of Southern California, Keck School of Medicine, 150 North Robertson Boulevard, Suite 314, Beverly Hills, CA 90211, USA
* Corresponding author.
E-mail address: gmassry@drmassry.com

upper blepharoplasty surgery by publishing on a more advanced anatomic knowledge of the upper lid, including the various fat compartments. Flowers[7] and Seigel[8,9] popularized tissue excision techniques that led to a high crease, large tarsal platform, and a generally hollow upper sulcus. This subtractive form of surgery was in vogue until the early part of this century when a paradigm shift from surgery based on tissue excision to one in which tissue (ie, muscle and fat) is preserved developed.[10,11] This shift is founded on the concept of recreating the fuller aesthetic of youth rather than the gaunt stigmata of the more traditional excision-based procedures.

This article reviews adjuncts to upper blepharoplasty that can be performed at the time of surgery to potentially enhance results. The techniques described are quick, minimally invasive, low-risk, and mostly focus on the concept of volume preservation. All procedures can be performed through the standard eyelid crease incision except for the external browpexy variant.

INTERNAL AND EXTERNAL BROWPEXY

Contemporary upper blepharoplasty requires an evaluation and assessment of the eyebrow and upper lid as an aesthetic unit. Because temporal brow ptosis is a common aging change that can add to upper eyelid lid fullness, stabilizing or lifting the outer brow has become an essential adjunct to aesthetic upper blepharoplasty.[12,13] Formal brow lifting procedures are invasive, costly, and potentially fraught with motor and sensory neurologic defects.[14–17] A browpexy, or brow suture suspension, is not a formal lift. It is a measured anchoring of brow tissue (muscle and/or fat) to the periosteum of the frontal bone (or bone itself) above the superior orbital rim. Its purpose is to provide stabilization or a slight lift to the outer brow in a minimally invasive way to allow

appropriate skin excision during blepharoplasty. It is typically added as an enhancement to blepharoplasty but also can be an isolated procedure.

The internal variant of the procedure was first described by McCord and Doxanas[13] in 1990. In this original description, the subbrow tissue is accessed through a blepharoplasty eyelid crease incision and the brow fat pad is dissected free of the frontal periosteum for variable distances from the orbital rim. A guiding suture can be placed from skin to the internal wound to ensure the appropriate placement of the suspension suture on the undersurface of the brow soft tissue. The area of brow suspension to the frontal bone periosteum is measured directly. A 4-0 Prolene (Ethicon, Somerville, NJ) or similar suture engages the periosteum at this location and also the internal brow tissue at the predetermined area (typically the inferior brow). Two to 3 similar sutures are placed laterally. When all sutures are tied, the brow is anchored to a new position.

Since its early description, there have been modifications of the procedure that have included extended dissection, release of deep retaining ligaments of the brow, extirpation of the temporal brow depressor muscle (lateral orbital orbicularis oculi), and the use of an external anchoring device fixated to the frontal bone (Endotine, Coapt Systems, Palo Alto, CA) (**Fig. 1**).[18–22] The main problem with all these procedures has been inconsistent results. Often no lift or stabilization was noted by surgeon or patient beyond a short-term result. This can be related to surgeon experience, technique, limitation of dissection, weakness of the procedure, or some combination thereof.

More recently, an external variant of this procedure has been described, which has been called the "External Browpexy".[23] In this variant, an 8 mm marking is made, tangential to the superior brow hairs or within the superior brow hairs, at the

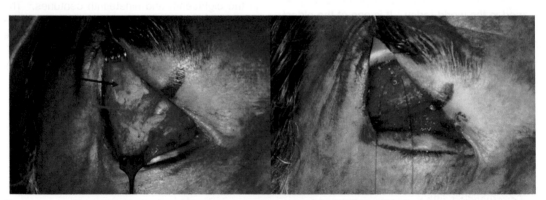

Fig. 1. Internal browpexy procedure. Left: Exposure of the brow fat pad above (*black arrow*) and the periosteum of the frontal bone below (*red arrow*). In the initial description of the internal browpexy, the fat pad is secured at a desired location to the periosteum. Right: Modification of procedure with implanted Endotine device.

junction of the body and tail of the brow. The exact location is determined in the preoperative area with the patient in the sitting position. The authors' preference has been to select an area at the superior brow that corresponds to a line drawn through the nasal ala and lateral limbus or pupil. The point is determined based on brow arch and lift desired, and can be modified depending on patient desires and gender. This area is elevated to the desired brow height. The marking pen is placed at this new height and the brow is allowed to return to its native position. A second mark is then made on the skin above the brow with the brow at this native position (Fig. 2). The distance between the 2 marks is the amount of lift to be achieved.

The procedure begins with a punch incision made to the periosteum at the demarcated area at the superior brow hairs. Whereas the external incision is small, the internal dissection proceeds medially and laterally to the periosteum for 25 mm (3× external incision). The basis for this is that the skin incision is small to lessen potential scarring but the internal dissection is larger for more raw surface area and subsequent cicatrix to anchor the brow. The periosteum at the level of the elevated brow height is then engaged with a forceps and a

4-0 Prolene suture on a P-3 needle is secured to the periosteum at this location. The suture is then passed from below, through the brow fat pad and orbicularis muscle, and then redirected from above through orbicularis muscle and the brow fat pad and tied. An elevation and anterior rotation of the brow is achieved. In addition, brow fullness may be recreated because the brow fat elevates and rotates similarly. The wound is then closed in layers (Figs. 3 and 4, Video 1 Part 1).

The senior author has performed this procedure on more than 100 patients during the last 4 years. The surgical results have been good, with rare minor and reversible complications. Specifically, there has been negligible scarring, no suture spitting or migration, no granulomas, and no infections or contour issues. A few patients have noted prolonged pain or tenderness over the brow suspension suture. These symptoms have resolved with time and/or serial injections of fluorouracil 50 mg/mL and/or Kenalog 5 mg/mL. The best measure of the potential for this procedure was noted in patients who presented with unilateral brow ptosis and had surgery only on that side to create symmetry. The authors have found a routine improvement in symmetry in these cases (Fig. 5). A current

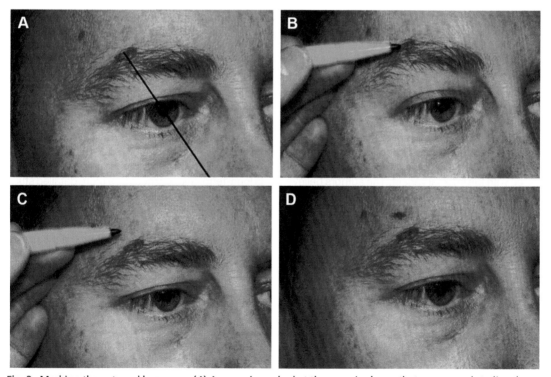

Fig. 2. Marking the external browpexy (A) An area is marked at the superior brow that corresponds to line drawn through the nasal ala and lateral limbus or midpupil. (B) This area is manually elevated to the desired brow height. The marking pen is placed hovering at this new height. (C) The brow is allowed to return to its native position. (D) A second mark is made on the skin above the brow at this native position. The distance between the 2 marks is the amount of lift to be achieved.

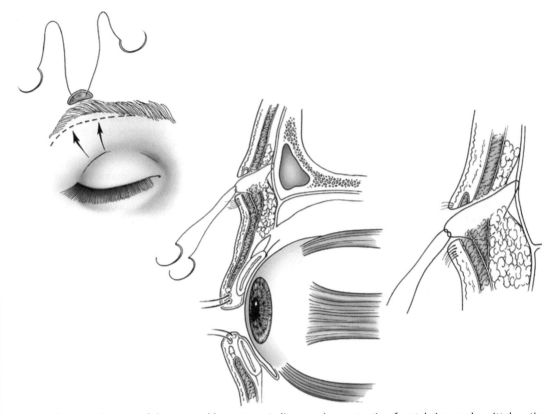

Fig. 3. Schematic drawing of the external browpexy. A diagram demonstrating frontal view and sagittal-section of the external browpexy suture. The suture tethers the brow fat pad and the frontalis-orbicularis interdigitation to the frontal bone periosteum at the desired height. The *arrows* simulate the vector of brow elevation. (*Adapted from* Massry GG. The external browpexy. Ophthal Plast Reconstr Surg 2012;28(2):90–5; with permission.)

ongoing study evaluating the results of this procedure has shown a mean brow elevation of 2.97 mm laterally and 1.90 mm centrally at an average 6 months follow-up.[24] Granted, these are short-term results, but they are encouraging and more substantial than what the authors have experienced with the internal variant. The authors believe the external procedure yields more reliable results than the internal technique because

1. There is lift from above rather than support from below
2. The superior fixation prevents the brow from pivoting over the anchor point
3. The orbicularis muscle and brow fat pad are anchored instead of just the fat pad
4. Brow elevation and suture placement are more precisely measured
5. The brow fat pad is elevated and anteriorly rotated, which may better volumetrically enhance the brow.

Of note, the idea for this procedure arose from observing patients who had traumatic full thickness (to bone) lacerations above the brow. It was observed that, in several of these patients, a localized peak (lift) in the brow developed after the wound healed. From this observation, the concept of a controlled suprabrow brow incision and fixation to bone developed. Overall, the authors have been pleased with this procedure. Whether there is long-term efficacy requires a more detailed study with serial standardized measurements of brow height over time. This is the next step in the continued evolution of the procedure. Most importantly, however, patients have been very satisfied with both the option of a noninvasive brow rejuvenation procedure and the surgical results.

NASAL FAT PRESERVATION/TRANSLOCATION UPPER BLEPHAROPLASTY

Hollowing of the upper eyelid and sulcus can occur as a normal consequence of aging or iatrogenically after traditional excisional (subtractive) blepharoplasty techniques.[25–27] Overzealous removal of skin, muscle, and fat often results in a gaunt or skeletonized appearance after surgery that is in contrast to the more contemporary understanding

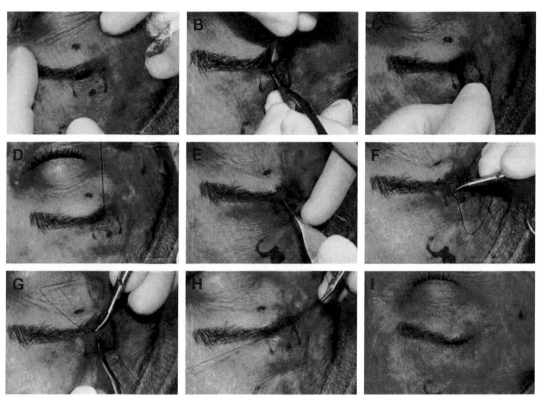

Fig. 4. Surgical series for the external browpexy. (*A*) Skin incision over demarcated area. (*B*) Frontalis-orbicularis division to periosteum. The internal dissection extends 3× the skin incision. (*C*) Periosteum engaged at predetermined area with forceps. (*D*) A 4-0 Prolene suture on a P-3 needle is used to engage the periosteum. (*E*) The orbicularis and brow fat are elevated. (*F*) The suture is passed from below, through the brow fat pad or orbicularis muscle. (*G*) The suture is redirected from above through the orbicularis muscle or brow fat pad. (*H*) The suture is tied, causing elevation of the brow. (*I*) The wound is closed in layers. (*From* Massry GG. The external browpexy. Ophthal Plast Reconstr Surg 2012;28(2):90–5; with permission.)

of the youthful fullness, curves, contours, and smooth topographic transitions of the eyebrow–upper eyelid aesthetic unit. This volume-depleted appearance unmasks the orbital rim, depletes the upper sulcus, and may lead to an A-frame deformity. Although the general tissue debulking inherent to this form of surgery can initially create a lighter and less puffy eyelid, patients invariably develop the typical volume-deficient stigmata of traditional upper blepharoplasty. These sequelae can be addressed with secondary interventions such as fat transfer,[28,29] grafts,[30–32] and injectable fillers.[33] However, appropriate preoperative evaluation and surgical planning may prevent these issues and the needed or secondary interventions.

Nasal fat pad translocation is a novel approach to upper blepharoplasty in which nasal upper eyelid/orbital fat is preserved and redistributed from areas of relative excess to areas of relative deficit. Such adjunctive fat pad preservation and translocation may lessen or prevent the volume-deficient results often seen with traditional

surgery. Similar techniques in lower blepharoplasty have gained wide acceptance as a normal adjunct to surgery that may more adequately address the transition of the lower eyelid to the cheek and prevent the postoperative volume loss associated with standard fat excision procedures.[34–36] Similar thinking, until recently, has lagged in regards to upper eyelid surgery. The authors have studied upper lid fat preservation techniques in detail and believe they are a better option to attaining the most appropriate long-term aesthetic surgical results.

The concept of preserving native upper eyelid fat in blepharoplasty surgery was not developed by the authors; it was modified from previously documented procedures. In 2010, Sozer and colleagues[37] reported on transposition of the central (preaponeurotic) eyelid fat to the temporal eyelid to create lateral fullness. The authors have little experience with this procedure and cannot comment on its utility. However, because the central eyelid fat tends toward involution with age,

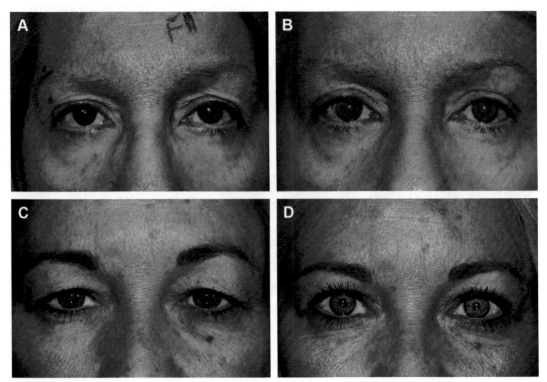

Fig. 5. Surgical results for the external browpexy. (*A*) Preoperative view of a patient with brow asymmetry and dermatochalasis with marks delineating the desired amount of brow elevation. (*B*) Postoperative result after right external browpexy and bilateral blepharoplasty. (*C*) Another patient with brow asymmetry and dermatochalasis. (*D*) Postoperative result after right external browpexy and bilateral upper lid blepharoplasty. These cases provide an assessment of procedure efficacy because the side not operated on acts a control. (*From* Massry GG. The external browpexy. Ophthal Plast Reconstr Surg 2012;28(2):90–5; with permission.)

there is concern that transposing this fat pedicle may advance central lid hollows and potential A-frame appearance. Park and colleagues[38] reported on combined inferior transposition of the nasal and central eyelid fat pads from the level of Whitnall ligament to the inferior eyelid, in the particular subset of Asian patients. They termed this procedure orbital fat relocation and thought it added to the fuller appearance of eyelids in these patients. In both reports, the investigators reported no complications with excellent surgical results.

The authors have focused attention on isolated transposition of nasal eyelid fat during blepharoplasty. There is evidence of the utility of such thinking. The nasal fat pad of the upper lid is anatomically, structurally, and clinically different than the central eyelid fat.[25] Nasal fat is whiter, denser, and continuous with deeper extraconal and intraconal orbital fat (**Fig. 6**). This is in contrast to the central eyelid fat compartment. This fat is less dense, yellower, and separated from deeper orbital fat by the levator aponeurosis. Therefore, the central fat pad is referred to as preaponeurotic. This is also why nasal upper eyelid fat can be accessed transconjunctivally (there is no aponeurosis to potentially damage).[39] The nasal fat pad has also been shown to be relatively stem cell–rich and to

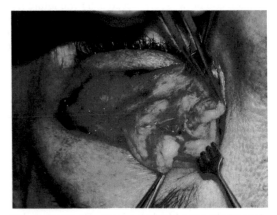

Fig. 6. Surgical anatomy of the upper eyelid fat pads. Upper right is forceps grasping the nasal fat pad. This fat is denser, yellower, and relatively stem cell–rich compared with the central eyelid fat. This fat is also in continuity with deeper orbital fat. Below center is forceps engaging the central eyelid fat. This fat is less dense, yellower, and relatively stem cell–poor. This fat is also called the preaponeurotic fat because it lies above the levator aponeurosis. Note the white aponeurosis below the fat pad. The aponeurosis attaches to the superomedial orbit around the nasal fat. The trochlea (pulley of the superior oblique tendon) lies deep between these fat pads. Special care must be placed at preserving the integrity of the trochlea during surgery.

clinically tend toward prominence with age. Conversely, the central eyelid fat is relatively stem cell–poor and, typically, clinically involves with age.[40,41] These eyelid fat pad characteristics are the basis of isolating a nasal fat pedicle for transfer in blepharoplasty surgery. The goal is to transpose stem cell–rich and clinically prominent eyelid fat from areas of excess to areas of deficit.

The variations of nasal fat transposition in blepharoplasty are (1) within the eyelid proper (**Fig. 7**)[25] and (2) outside of the eyelid proper (**Figs. 8 and 9**).[27] The initial surgical steps for each are similar. The procedures only differ in where the fat is placed. In both, a standard skin excision blepharoplasty is performed. The nasal and central orbicularis muscle and orbital septum are divided to access the nasal and central fat compartments. The nasal fat is freed of all connective tissue attachments to surrounding structures so that it becomes a freely mobile fat flap. In this step it is critical to be wary of the superior oblique tendon and trochlea that separate the fat pads of the upper lid (akin to the inferior oblique muscle in the lower lid).[42] Damage to these structures can lead to postoperative diplopia (pseudo-Brown syndrome).[43] This occurred to the authors once early on and resolved with local steroid injection and time. Also, if the nasal pedicle is not freely mobile when it is transposed centrally, it can potentially place pressure on the levator aponeurosis and lead to transient ptosis (also seen in a few early cases). When nasal fat is transposed within the eyelid, the fat flap is secured to the superior orbital rim periosteum, undersurface of the orbital septum, or the orbicularis muscle in the central eyelid. The fat is draped loosely, which is confirmed by elevating it off of the aponeurosis

to ensure lack of tension on underlying structures (see Video 1 Part 2).

When fat is transposed outside of the eyelid, it is placed over a depression at the superonasal orbital rim. The authors call this hollow the orbito-glabellar groove (OGG) because of its adjacent anatomic structures.[27] This depression is in continuity with the nasojugal groove (tear trough) at the nasal lower lid-cheek interface and cannot be effaced with standard blepharoplasty surgery. In fact, it is often worsened with the traditional surgical approach. In this procedure, a preperiosteal dissection begins below the OGG until a continuous pocket is created. The nasal fat flap (fashioned as previously described) is transposed to this pocket with a full-thickness transcutaneous suture. The filling effect of the fat smooths the medial brow upper lid transition (see Video 1 Part 3). After fat transposition in both procedures, the skin is closed in the usual way. **Fig. 10** depicts typical results of both fat preservation techniques.

LACRIMAL GLAND REPOSITIONING

A dislocated lacrimal gland can add to temporal fullness of the eyelid.[20] It can be clinically seen by having the patient look down and watching for fullness to the temporal eyelid below the superior orbital rim (**Fig. 11**). This fullness presents as a mass effect and is freely mobile without adherence to surrounding tissue. Lacrimal gland prolapse (LGP) was traditionally suggested to be clinically evident in 15% of patients presenting for blepharoplasty.[44,45] In a recent study, it was identified intraoperatively in up to 60% of subjects undergoing functional upper lid blepharoplasty.[46] In the same report LGP was subdivided into mild 24%

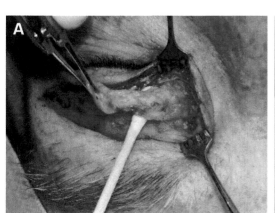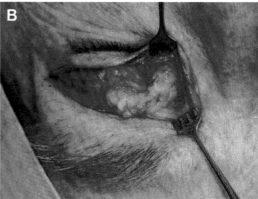

Fig. 7. Nasal fat pad translocation within the eyelid. (*A*) The nasal fat pad (over cotton-tip applicator) is isolated and mobilized as a free fat pedicle. (*B*)The nasal fat pad is then draped over the levator aponeurosis and central fat pad and secured to the central eyelid. (*From* Massry GG. Nasal fat preservation in upper eyelid blepharoplasty. Ophthal Plast Reconstr Surg 2011;27():352–5; with permission.)

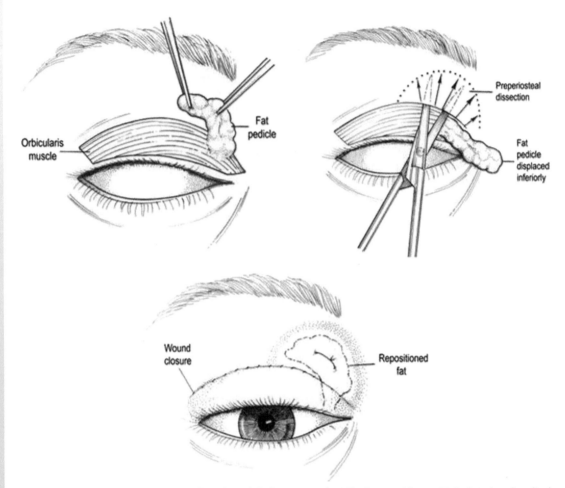

Fig. 8. Nasal fat pad translocation to the orbitoglabellar groove (OGG). The nasal fat pad is isolated and pedicalized. It is then translocated superiorly into a preperiosteal pocket underlying the OGG (volume deficient area). (*From* Yoo DB, Peng G, Massry GG. Effacing the orbitoglabellar groove with transposed upper eyelid fat. Ophthal Plast Reconstr Surg 2013;29(3):220–4; with permission.)

(0–2 mm from orbital rim), moderate 67% (3–5 mm from orbital rim), and severe 9% (6 mm or more from orbital rim). The study suggested that LGP, like dermatochalasis, relative fat herniation, and ptosis is most likely a normal involutional eyelid/ orbital change. It is not known whether repositioning a prolapsed lacrimal gland improves surgical outcome cosmetically because there has been no controlled study evaluating this question. However, it intuitively makes sense that a severe prolapse would benefit from repositioning to reduce the temporal bulge. It is also important to note that in the upper lid, although central eyelid fat often is displaced laterally, there is no distinct lateral fat pad (as in the lower lid). It is important to not inadvertently resect the lacrimal gland with the mistaken thought that it is lateral eyelid fat.

LGP has been managed with segmental resection,[44] suture repositioning,[20,45,47] and light cautery.[46] Lacrimal gland resection is now uncommon

and suture suspension is the norm. In mild or moderate prolapse, the authors typically apply light cautery to shrink the gland capsule and superficial parenchyma. This tends to retroplace the gland by creating a cicatrix, which obviates a suture. This step is quick, simple, and avoids the occasional bleeding encountered with suture suspension of the gland. The authors are unsure whether the damage created from cauterizing the tip of the gland and its capsule is any different from the injury associated with suture suspension from tissue penetration with the suture and strangulation when the knot is tied.

Lacrimal gland suture suspension is generally straightforward. The prolapsed gland is identified. The gland has a pale color with obvious glandular elements that are distinctly different than the clinical appearance of adjacent fat (**Fig. 12**). A 5-0 Prolene suture on a P-3 needle engages the gland capsule. The suture is then secured to the anterior tip of the lacrimal gland fossa periosteum

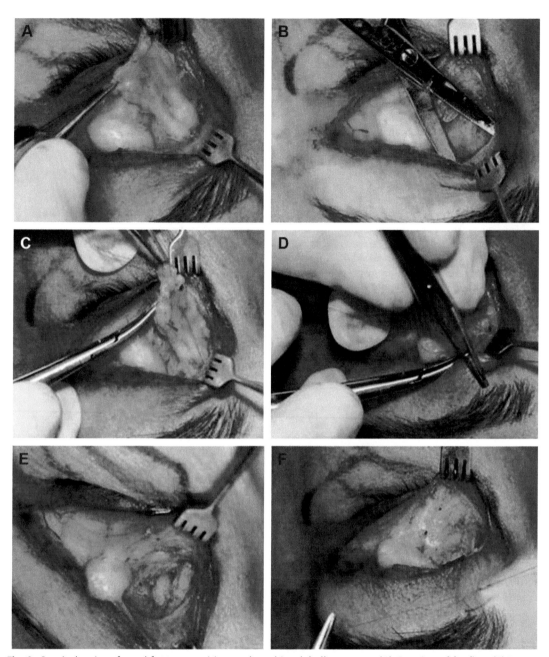

Fig. 9. Surgical series of nasal fat transposition to the orbitoglabellar groove. (*A*) Creation of fat flap. (*B*) Preperiosteal dissection of pocket for fat repositioning. (*C*) Engaging fat flap. (*D*) Transcutaneous fixation of fat flap. (*E*) Fat flap in preperiosteal pocket. (*F*) Suture tied. (*From* Yoo DB, Peng G, Massry GG. Effacing the orbitoglabellar groove with transposed upper eyelid fat. Ophthal Plast Reconstr Surg 2013;29(3):220–4; with permission.)

at the superior orbital rim. This returns the gland to its normal anatomic location (see Video 1 Part 4). The eyelid is then closed in the standard fashion.

BRASSIERE SUTURE FIXATION OF BROW FAT PAD

Browpexy techniques to elevate or stabilize the temporal eyebrow were previously discussed.

Here we review a technique to elevate (reposition) the brow fat pad to a position at, or above, the orbital rim to add a more youthful fullness and contour to the lateral brow. The eyebrow is a complex structure similar to the eyelid in that it is anatomically composed of multiple lamellae that include skin, muscle, connective tissue elements, and fat.[23] The fat compartment of the eyebrow is the brow fat pad or retroorbicularis oculi fat. It is

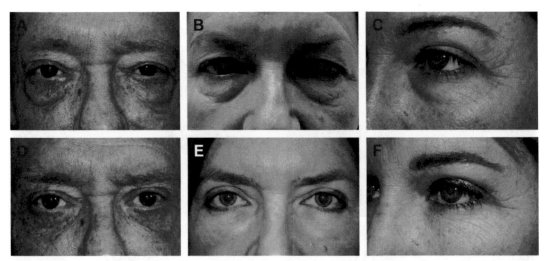

Fig. 10. Clinical results of 3 patients who underwent upper blepharoplasty with nasal fat transposition. The preoperative photograph is above and the postoperative result below in each case. (*A, B*) Nasal fat preservation (translocation) was planned within the eyelid proper prior to upper blepharoplasty. (*D, E*) Postoperative results at 1-year follow-up. There is no evidence of sulcus hollowing. (*C*) Preoperative view of OGG depression prior to upper blepharoplasty. (*F*) On oblique view it is seen that the OGG has been effaced significantly with improved contour. (*Adapted from* Yoo DB, Peng G, Massry GG. Effacing the orbitoglabellar groove with transposed upper eyelid fat. Ophthal Plast Reconstr Surg 2013;29(3):220–4; with permission.)

encased above and below by the anterior and posterior leafs of the deep layer of galea aponeurotica, and lies just above the periosteum of the frontal bone.[20] In white patients, the brow fat continues into the eyelids as the postorbicular fascial plane[48] and, in Asian patients, as the preseptal fat layer.[49,50] Like the brow proper, normal aging causes the brow fat pad to descend, sometimes below the orbital rim. In addition, the brow fat tends toward age-related deflation (volume loss).

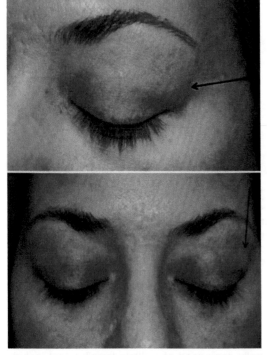

Fig. 11. Lacrimal gland prolapse. A dislocated lacrimal gland causes fullness that presents as a mass effect and is freely mobile without adherence to surrounding tissue (*arrows*).

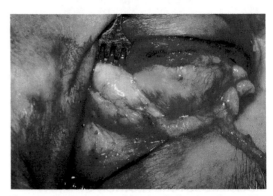

Fig. 12. Surgical view of lacrimal gland prolapse. The prolapsed gland has a pale color with obvious glandular elements. This is distinctly different than the clinical appearance of adjacent fat.

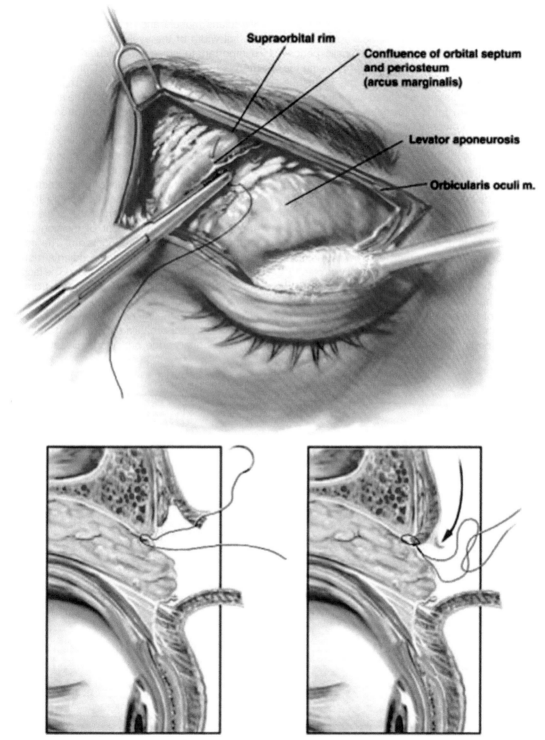

Fig. 13. Dr Zarem's drawings of brow fat suspension suture. Note the suture is fixated to the superior orbital rim arcus marginalis and then to the orbicularis muscle at the superior wound edge. (*From* Zarem HA. Browpexy. Aesthet Surg J 2004;24(4):368–72; with permission.)

In 1997, Zarem and colleagues[51] described an upper blepharoplasty variant in which the orbicularis muscle at the upper edge of the blepharoplasty incision is secured the arcus marginalis periosteum at the superior orbital rim before closing the skin incision. Dr Zarem presented this technique as a means to create a defined superior sulcus (especially when fat is excised) and support the outer brow (browpexy variant). The procedure was described again by Zarem[52] in 2003 (**Fig. 13**). During the last 4 years, the authors have used their version of this suspension suture procedure. This version was initially described to the authors by an oculofacial surgeon (Jonathan Hoeing, MD, personal communication, 2008). The authors think the technique's primary focus is to elevate and suspend the brow fat pad. In essence, it creates a barrier for brow fat descent and bunches the brow fat, potentially projecting it anteriorly (a form of volume enhancement). This variation has been called the brassiere suture suspension of the brow fat pad because it supports and lifts the brow fat in a fashion similar to a brassiere supporting ptotic breast tissue.

After standard blepharoplasty skin excision, the orbicularis muscle and orbital septum is opened the full width of the eyelid (nasal to temporal). It is important to incise the orbicularis muscle along the center of the eyelid defect and to leave an equal amount of free orbicularis muscle above and below the skin wound edges. The authors prefer to slip the wooden end of a cotton-tip applicator below the septum and muscle and slide it to the temporal end of the incision. The applicator is then elevated, tenting up the septum and muscle. A cut down is then performed directly on the applicator. This allows a level of protection for the levator aponeurosis; delineates the incision on the muscle; and, by altering the angle of the applicator, allows adjustment of incision placement (to assure a centered incision). The central fat pad is teased free from surrounding structures so that the lateral orbital rim is in view. The lacrimal gland, if present, is bluntly separated from the orbital rim periosteum. Two 5-0 chromic sutures are placed from the inferior wound edge orbicularis to the superior orbital rim periosteum and to the superior wound edge orbicularis. Because equal

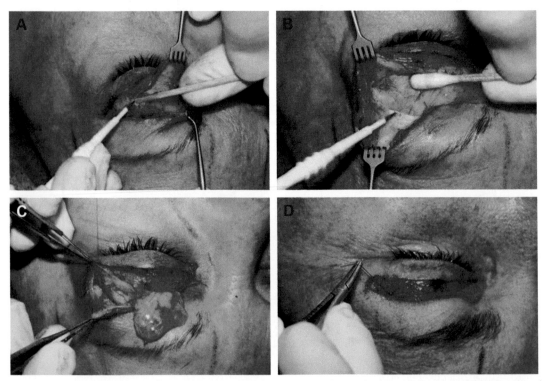

Fig. 14. Surgical series of brassiere suture technique. (*A*) The wooden end of a cotton-tip applicator is placed below the septum and orbicularis muscle and slid to the temporal end of the blepharoplasty incision. The applicator is then elevated, tenting up the septum and muscle. The muscle and septum are then divided over the applicator in the center of the wound using monopolar cautery. (*B*) Rakes splaying open wound with Colorado tip on arcus marginalis periosteum and cotton tip over aponeurosis. (*C*) Two 5-0 chromic sutures are placed from inferior wound edge orbicularis, orbital rim periosteum (see Colorado tip in *B*), and superior wound edge orbicularis. (*D*) The sutures are tied, supporting and projecting the brow fat pad anteriorly.

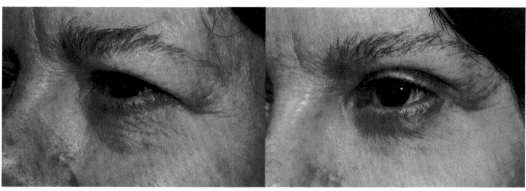

Fig. 15. Clinical result of brassiere suture fixation of brow fat pad. A woman before (*left*) and after (*right*) temporal endoscopic brow lift and brassiere suture fat pad suspension. Note the fullness of brow and delineation of the temporal eyelid crease.

orbicularis muscle is designed from above and below the muscle cut, orbicularis anchoring to the orbital rim is centered (**Fig. 14**). The authors think this may prevent a mechanical limitation of eyelid elevation (an initial concern), which has not manifested as a postoperative issue with the technique described (see Video 1 Part 5). The eyelid wound is then closed in the standard fashion. The authors have noted excellent surgical results (improved brow fullness, contour, and delineation of temporal eyelid crease) without more than minor and transient complications (**Fig. 15**).

SUMMARY

In an ongoing effort to improve results to upper blepharoplasty surgery, a variety of minimally invasive surgical adjuncts have been described. This article focuses on written, photographic, and video-assisted descriptions of these various techniques. Most of the procedures emphasize volume preservation and are performed through an eyelid crease incision (with the exception of the external browpexy). The authors suggest a basic framework of understanding of these interventions because they can enhance surgical outcomes and improve patient satisfaction.

SUPPLEMENTARY DATA

Supplementary data related to this article can be found online at http://dx.doi.org/10.1016/j.fsc. 2015.01.013.

REFERENCES

1. Lee JW, Baker SR. Esthetic enhancements in upper blepharoplasty. In: Azizzadeh B, Massry GG, editors-. Clinics in plastic surgery: brow and upper eyelid surgery: multispecialty approach. Clin Plast Surg 2013;40:139–46.

2. Adamson P, Moran M. Historical trends in surgery for the aging face. Facial Plast Surg 1993;9:133–42.

3. Wolfort FG, Colon F, Wolfort S, et al. The history of blepharoplasty. In: Wolfort FG, Kanroe WR, editors. Aesthetic blepharoplasty. Boston: Little Brown; 1995. p. 1–16.

4. Wood C. The tadhkirat of ali ibn isa of baghdad (transl). Chicago: Northwestern University; 1936. p. 98, 115, 118–119.

5. Dupris C, Rees TD. Historical notes on blepharoplasty. Plast Reconstr Surg 1971;47:246–51.

6. Costaneras S. Blepharoplasty for herniated intraorbital fat: anatomic basis for a new approach. Plast Reconstr Surg 1951;8:46.

7. Flowers RS. Upper blepharoplasty by eyelid invagination: anchor blepharoplasty. Clin Plast Surg 1993; 20:193–207.

8. Siegel RJ. Essential anatomy of contemporary upper lid blepharoplasty. Clin Plast Surg 1993;20: 209–12.

9. Siegel RJ. Contemporary upper lid blepharoplasty. Tissue invagination. Clin Plast Surg 1993; 20:239–46.

10. Fagien S. Advanced rejuvenative upper blepharoplasty: enhancing aesthetics of the upper periorbita. Plast Reconstr Surg 2002;110:278–92.

11. Kulbersh JS, Massry GG, Azizzadeh BA. Periorbital aesthetic surgery: the evolution. Of a multidisciplinary surgical specialty. In: Massry GG, Murphy MR, Azizzadeh B, editors. Master techniques in blepharoplasty and periorbital rejuvenation. New York: Springer; 2011. p. 3–10.

12. Georgescu D, Anderson RL, McCann JD. Brow ptosis correction: a comparison of five techniques. Facial Plast Surg 2010;26:186–92.

13. McCord CD, Doxanas MT. Browplasty and browpexy: an adjunct to blepharoplasty. Plast Reconstr Surg 1990;86:248–54.

14. Paul MD. The evolution of the brow lift in aesthetic plastic surgery. Plast Reconstr Surg 2001;108:1409–24.

15. Green JP, Goldberg RA, Shorr N. Eyebrow ptosis. Int Ophthalmol Clin 1997;37:97–122.

16. Keller GS, Hutcherson RW. Browlift: a facial plastic surgeon's perspective. In: Romo T III, Millman AL, editors. Aesthetic facial plastic surgery—a multidisciplinary approach. New York: Thieme; 2000. p. 226–35.

17. Wojtanowski MH. Bicoronal forehead lift. Aesthetic Plast Surg 1994;18:33–9.

18. Burroughs JR, Bearden WH, Anderson RL, et al. Internal brow elevation at blepharoplasty. Arch Facial Plast Surg 2006;8:36–41.

19. Tyers AG. Brow lift via the direct and trans-blepharoplasty approaches. Orbit 2006;25:261–5.

20. Georgescu D, Belsare G, McCann JD, et al. Adjunctive procedures in upper eyelid blepharoplasty: internal brow fat sculpting and elevation, glabellar myectomy, and lacrimal gland repositioning. In: Massry GG, Murphy MR, Azizzadeh B, editors. Master techniques in blepharoplasty and periorbital rejuvenation. New York: Springer; 2011. p. 101–8.

21. Niechajev I. Transpalpebral browpexy. Plast Reconstr Surg 2004;113:2172–80.

22. Cohen BD, Reiffel AJ, Spinelli HM. Browpexy through the upper lid (BUL): a new technique of lifting the brow with a standard blepharoplasty incision. Aesthet Surg J 2011;31:163–9.

23. Massry G. The external browpexy. Ophthal Plast Reconstr Surg 2012;28(2):90–5.

24. Mokhtarzadeh A, Harrison A, Massry G. Quantitative efficacy of internal and external browpexy. Annual spring meeting of the American Society of Ophthalmic Plastic and Reconstructive Surgery. Park City (Utah), June 2014.

25. Massry G. Nasal fat preservation in upper eyelid blepharoplasty. Ophthal Plast Reconstr Surg 2011; 27:352–5.

26. Massry G. Commentary on "the sigmoidal upper blepharoplasty". Ophthal Plast Reconstr Surg 2012;28:454.

27. Yoo DB, Peng G, Massry G. Effacing the orbitoglabellar groove with transposed upper eyelid fat. Ophthal Plast Reconstr Surg 2013;29:220–4.

28. Glasgold RA, Lam SM, Glasgold MJ. Periorbital fat grafting. In: Massry GG, Azizzadeh B, Murphy M, editors. Master techniques in blepharoplasty and periorbital rejuvenation. New York: Springer; 2011. p. 259–72.

29. Massry G, Azizzadeh B. Periorbital fat grafting. Facial Plast Surg 2013;29:46–57.

30. Czyz C, Lam VB, Foster JA. Management of complications of upper eyelid blepharoplasty. In: Massry GG, Murphy MR, Azizzadeh B, editors. Master techniques in blepharoplasty and periorbital rejuvenation. New York: Springer; 2011. p. 109–23.

31. Fezza JP. The sigmoid upper eyelid blepharoplasty: redefining beauty. Ophthal Plast Reconstr Surg 2012;28:446–51.

32. Glasgold RA, Glasgold MJ. The sigmoid upper eyelid blepharoplasty: commentary. Ophthal Plast Reconstr Surg 2012;28:452–3.

33. Morley AM, Taban M, Malhotra R, et al. Use of hyaluronic Acid gel for upper eyelid filling and contouring. Ophthal Plast Reconstr Surg 2009;25:440–4.

34. Hamra ST. The role of orbital fat preservation in facial aesthetic surgery. A new concept. Clin Plast Surg 1996;23:17–28.

35. Goldberg RA. Transconjunctival orbital fat repositioning: transposition of orbital fat pedicles into a subperiosteal pocket. Plast Reconstr Surg 2000; 105:743–8.

36. Massry GG. Comprehensive lower eyelid rejuvenation. Facial Plast Surg 2010;26:209–21.

37. Sozer SO, Agullo FJ, Palladino H, et al. Pedicle fat flap to increase lateral fullness in upper blepharoplasty. Aesthet Surg J 2010;30(2):161–5.

38. Park SK, Kim BG, Shin YH. Correction of superior sulcus deformity with orbital fat anatomic repositioning and fat graft applied to retroorbicularis oculi fat for Asian eyelids. Aesthetic Plast Surg 2011;35: 162–70. Available at: http://www.springerlink.

39. Nahai F. Transconjunctival upper lid blepharoplasty. Aesthet Surg J 2005;25:292–300.

40. Korn BS, Kikkawa DO, Hicok KC. Identification and characterization of adult stem cells from human orbital adipose tissue. Ophthal Plast Reconstr Surg 2009;25:27–32.

41. Sang-Rog O, Weerawan C, Annunziata CC, et al. Paper Presentation. ASOPRS Fall Scientific Symposium. San Francisco (CA), October 21, 2009.

42. Tan KS, Oh SR, Priel A, et al. Surgical anatomy of the forehead, eyelids and midface for the aesthetic surgeon. In: Massry GG, Murphy MR, Azizzadeh B, editors. Master techniques in blepharoplasty and periorbital rejuvenation. New York: Springer; 2011. p. 11–24.

43. Neely KA, Ernest JT, Mottier M. Combined superior oblique paresis and Brown's syndrome after blepharoplasty. Am J Ophthalmol 1990;109(3):347–9.

44. Smith B, Lisman RD. Dacryoadenopexy as a recognized factor in upper lid blepharoplasty. Plast Reconstr Surg 1983;71:629–32.

45. Beer GM, Kompatscher P. A new technique for the treatment of lacrimal gland prolapse in blepharoplasty. Aesthetic Plast Surg 1994;18:65–9.

46. Massry G. Prevalence of lacrimal gland prolapse in the functional blepharoplasty population. Ophthal Plast Reconstr Surg 2011;27:410–3.

47. Smith B, Petrelli R. Surgical repair of prolapsed lacrimal glands. Arch Ophthalmol 1978;96:1132.

48. Putterman AM, Urist MJ. Surgical anatomy of the orbital septum. Ann Ophthalmol 1974;6:290–4.

49. Meyer DR, Linberg JV, Wobig JL. Anatomy of the orbital septum and associated eyelid connective tissues. Implications for ptosis surgery. Ophthal Plast Reconstr Surg 1991;7:104–13.

50. Seiff SR, Seiff BD. Anatomy of the Asian eyelid. Facial Plast Surg Clin North Am 2007;15:309–14.

51. Zarem HA, Resnick JI, Carr RM, et al. Browpexy: lateral orbicularis muscle fixation as an adjunct to upper blepharoplasty. Plast Reconstr Surg 1997; 100:1258–61.

52. Zarem HA. Browpexy. Aesthet Surg J 2004;24: 368–72.

Minimally Invasive Options for the Brow and Upper Lid

César A. Briceño, MD[a], Sandy X. Zhang-Nunes, MD[b], Guy G. Massry, MD[c],*

KEYWORDS

- Brow • Upper eyelid • Eyebrow anatomy • Eyelid anatomy • Fillers • Neuromodulators
- Facial aging

KEY POINTS

- Aging of the brow and upper eyelid occurs in all tissue planes and involves cutaneous changes, volume loss, and tissue descent.
- Volume restoration and neuromodulation have become an integral part of eyebrow/eyelid aesthetic rejuvenation.
- Surgical lifting techniques alone, without addressing volume loss, are insufficient to address aging of the brow/upper eyelid complex.
- Preservation and restoration of skin quality can have dramatic rejuvenating effects to the brow and upper eyelid.

INTRODUCTION

Appropriate aesthetic rejuvenation of the eyelids and periorbital soft tissues requires a detailed knowledge of relevant anatomy and normal aging changes, and techniques to comprehensively address the presenting deficits and attain natural results to treatment. It has long been accepted that changes in skin quality and appearance and tissue descent convey obvious signs of aging and are principal players in this process. Surgical procedures to elevate and remove excess tissue have traditionally been considered the preferred means to address tissue sagging. Chemical denervation (neuromodulation; Botox botulinum toxin A [BoNTA]) has allowed the addition of effacing hyperdynamic lines and has been shown to be an excellent adjunct to surgery.[1] Over the past few decades, a paradigm shift has occurred, in which it has become clear that facial aging is a more complex, three-dimensional process, affecting all tissue planes (skin, muscle, fat, and bone).[2] The importance of the role of volume loss in this intricate process has been particularly emphasized,[1–7] especially in relation to the eyelids and periorbita.[7–12] As facial aging has been evaluated from the perspective of both tissue descent and deflation, more acceptable outcomes to treatment, both surgical and nonsurgical, have emerged.[8–12] As of 2011, statistics from the American Society of Plastic Surgery show that injection of BoNTA remains the single most performed cosmetic procedure in the United States (approximately 2.6 million procedures).[13] Also, the potential for restoring a youthful shape and contour to a patient's face has made fillers the fastest growing

[a] Department of Ophthalmology and Visual Sciences, Kellogg Eye Center, University of Michigan, 1000 Wall Street, Ann Arbor, MI 48105, USA; [b] Department of Ophthalmology, USC Eye Institute, Keck School of Medicine, University of Southern California, 1450 San Pablo Street, 4th floor, Los Angeles, CA 90033, USA; [c] Ophthalmic Plastic and Reconstructive Surgery, Keck School of Medicine, University of Southern California, 150 North Robertson Boulevard, Suite 314, Beverly Hills, CA 90211, USA
* Corresponding author.
E-mail address: gmassry@drmassry.com

Facial Plast Surg Clin N Am 23 (2015) 153–166
http://dx.doi.org/10.1016/j.fsc.2015.01.012
1064-7406/15/$ – see front matter © 2015 Elsevier Inc. All rights reserved.

facialplastic.theclinics.com

minimally invasive cosmetic procedure in the United States.[14] In 2011, about 1.2 million facial filling procedures involving hyaluronic acid (HA) were performed, constituting 84% of all filler procedures, and BoNTA and HA together comprise 75% of all nonsurgical procedures performed.[13] These data underscore the importance of contemporary minimally invasive methods of facial rejuvenation. Sundaram and Kiripolsky[15] described their means of addressing facial aging with an outcome-based approach to treatment. They called this the 4 pillars of rejuvenation. This approach includes (1) replacement of tissue volume, (2) regeneration of tissue quality, (3) rebalancing of facial vectors and proportions, and (4) improvement of skin reflectance. Minimally invasive techniques designed to address these principles have become core adjuncts to modern aesthetic facial rejuvenation and have allowed practitioners a means of attaining natural outcomes while avoiding the stigma of volume loss and hollowing associated with older reductive surgical techniques. This article focuses on minimally invasive options to rejuvenate the brow and upper lid complex, with a review of the relevant anatomy and contemporary concepts in upper facial aging.

EYEBROW/EYELID ANATOMY

Although a detailed description of anatomic considerations of the eyebrow and eyelid is beyond the scope of this article, a general understanding of the relevant structures of significance and how they transition from the brow to the eyelid is important. The eyebrow is a multilayered structure composed of cilia, skin, muscle, fat, and connective tissue elements.[16] The skin is thicker than that of the eyelid, which is important when manipulating the brow/lid transition. The paired frontalis muscles are the elevators of the eyebrow and originate from the galea aponeurotica, span the forehead from superior temporal line (STL) to STL, and insert on the skin (no bone insertion) at the superior brow after interdigitating with various muscle groups.[17] These muscle include the orbital orbicularis oculi muscle laterally, and the orbicularis oculi, procerus, and corrugator supercilii muscle medially (**Fig. 1**).[6,17] Although the frontalis is the only elevator of the eyebrows, the orbital

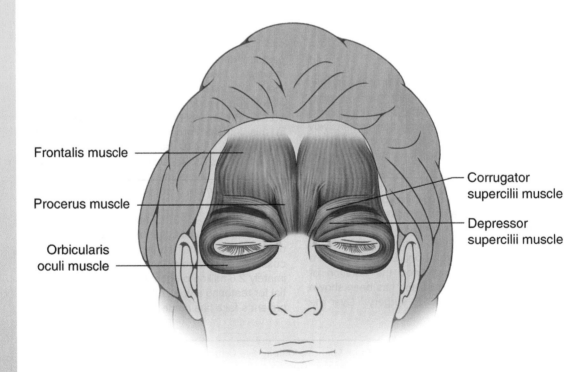

Fig. 1. Muscles that elevate and depress the eyebrows. Note the frontalis (brow elevator), and the orbital orbicularis, corrugator, and procerus muscles (brow depressors). The frontalis has no bone attachment and indirectly inserts into the skin after interdigitating with the brow depressor muscles. (*From* Tan KS, Oh SR, Priel A, et al. Surgical anatomy of the forehead, eyelids, and midface for the aesthetic surgeon. In: Massry GG, Murphy MR, Azizzadeh B, editors. Master techniques in blepharoplasty and periorbital rejuvenation. New York: Springer; 2011. p. 11–24; with permission.)

orbicularis, corrugator supercilii, and procerus muscles all depress the brow. There is no eyebrow elevator lateral to the STL, which makes this location especially prone to brow ptosis with age.[6]

The frontalis muscle is positioned between the superficial and deep layers of the galea aponeurotica proper.[16,18] Inferiorly, the deep layer of the galea splits into an anterior and posterior leaf that encase the retro-orbicularis oculi fat (ROOF) or brow fat pad.[16,18] Posterior to the ROOF is the periosteum of the frontal bone. The orbicularis retaining ligament (ORL) is an oseocutaneous structure arising from just above the orbital rim and inserting into the dermis of the skin. Laterally the ORL contributes to the lateral orbital thickening.[6] In combination, these structures lend a degree of support to the soft tissues of the eyebrows. At the superior orbital rim the periosteum of the frontal bone and orbit meet forming the arcus marginalis, which continues into the eyelid as the orbital septum.[19] The ROOF transitions into the eyelid as the postorbicularis fascial plane in caucasian people[20] and the preseptal fat layer in Asian people.[21,22] The orbital orbicularis from above continues into the eyelid as the preseptal and then pretarsal segments of the muscle (named according the structures they overlie).[19] Posterior to the orbital septum lie the nasal and central (preaponeurotic) fat compartments. The nasal fat pad is contiguous with the deeper orbital fat.[19,23,24] The preaponeurotic fat is separated from the deeper orbit by the levator aponeurosis.[19,23,24] The aponeurosis is an extension of the levator muscle, which is the primary upper eyelid retractor (elevator). The orbital septum overlies orbital fat and inserts onto the levator aponeurosis which then sends projections to the eyelid skin to form the eyelid crease.[25] The crease typically measures 7 to 8 mm from the lid margin in men and 10 mm in women. Posterior to the aponeurosis is the second eyelid elevator, the Müller muscle. This muscle is an autonomically innervated muscle that arises from the undersurface of the levator muscle and inserts onto the superior border of the tarsus (**Fig. 2**).[25]

RELEVANT TOPOGRAPHY OF THE YOUTHFUL AND AGED UPPER EYELID/BROW COMPLEX

The topography of the brow and upper eyelid vary according to gender, age, and ethnicity.[15] Common among all youthful brow/upper lid complexes is a three-dimensional structure with smooth curves and contours that transition well and reflect light in a natural way (**Fig. 3**).[6] With aging, changes in natural contour, related to tissue descent and deflation, cause these reflections to become

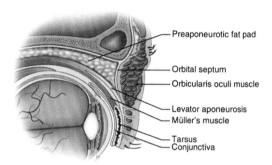

Fig. 2. Relevant anatomic structures of the upper eyelid. (*From* Morton AD. Upper eyelid blepharoplasty. In: Massry GG, Murphy MR, Azizzadeh B, editors. Master techniques in blepharoplasty and periorbital rejuvenation. New York: Springer; 2011. p. 87–100; with permission.)

interrupted, leading to associated shadowing (**Fig. 4**).[6] What underlies these involutional changes involves both static and dynamic components. The brow fat pad attenuates with age. In addition, there are equally significant involutional changes in bone, leading to loss of underlying support of the brow. This global loss of volume reduces the static support of the eyebrow, which often leads to secondary tissue descent. This concept of brow position and its relation to volume loss became obvious to one of us (GM) many years ago, because it was noted (also by many colleagues) that the injection of local anesthesia during facial surgery led to an immediate correction of some degree of tissue ptosis. These kinds of observations have led to the more contemporary

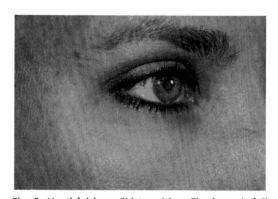

Fig. 3. Youthful brow/lid transition. The brow is full and transitions to the upper eyelid smoothly without obvious contour irregularities or shadowing. (*From* Buchanan AG, Holds JB. The beautiful eye: perception of beauty in the periocular area. In: Massry GG, Murphy MR, Azizzadeh B, editors. Master techniques in blepharoplasty and periorbital rejuvenation. New York: Springer; 2011. p. 25–30; with permission.)

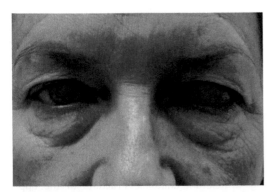

Fig. 4. The aged brow. With age the brow deflates and descends, leading to contour irregularities, lateral hooding, and shadowing. (*From* Massry GG, Nassif PS. Transconjunctival lower blepharoplasty: fat excision or repositioning. In: Massry GG, Murphy MR, Azizzadeh B, editors. Master techniques in blepharoplasty and periorbital rejuvenation. New York: Springer; 2011. p. 173–84; with permission.)

approach of volume augmentation facial/eyelid restorative surgery, and nonsurgical interventions.

In addition to volume, resting muscle tone is a critical component of typical brow/eyelid aging changes. This muscle tone is the dynamic component characteristic of eyebrow aging. As stated earlier, the frontalis muscle is the elevator of the eyebrows, and it spans the forehead from STL to STL. Temporal to the STL (approximately the junction of the body and tail of the brow) there is no brow elevator.[6,19] However, there is a depressor of the lateral brow, the orbital orbicularis muscle, lateral to the STL. Age and loss of static support shifts the dynamic equilibrium of brow position to unopposed descent. Consequently it is the lateral brow that tends to become ptotic with age, with the resultant characteristic lateral eyelid hooding for which so many patients seek correction (see **Fig. 4**). Although it is important to understand what underlies typical age-related outer brow ptosis, this should not be considered in isolation. Each patient is different and can present with different findings. The literature is not clear as to what happens to overall brow position with age, with data showing elevation, stability, or depression.[6,26,27] Again, this is a static and dynamic process in which the clinical manifestations may be compensatory (ie, the brow may elevate with age as a compensatory response to lid ptosis).[25]

The eyelids also show characteristic changes with age. The youthful lid is full and wide. Like the brow, it is devoid of depressions and contour irregularities.[28] With age there are characteristic changes in volume, both of the underlying bone and of soft tissue.[6] The orbit tends primarily to

remodel superonasally and inferotemporally.[29] This remodeling leads to loss of support in those areas and a rounder, more vertically oriented palpebral aperture. Canthal tendon laxity with medialization of the lateral canthus can exacerbate this change. As the eyelid loses soft tissue volume the upper eyelid skin becomes redundant, with both true and pseudoexcess, which leads to hanging skin and hollows. The hollows are most prominent centrally and nasally where the characteristic A-frame deformity occurs (**Fig. 5**).[6,23] In some patients with very devolumized orbits/eyelids, rather than skin sagging, the skin retracts into the upper sulcus, unmasking the pretarsal eyelid and giving a skeletonized appearance. When involutional ptosis is present this becomes even more obvious (see **Fig. 5**). In either instance the primary issue is loss of volume and support.

There are distinct differences between the appearance and topography of the male and female eyebrow. In both genders the brow begins medially in a line perpendicular to the medial canthus and nasal ala. It ends laterally in a line tangent to the nasal ala and lateral canthus. In addition, the medial and lateral brow lie vertically at the same level. The tail of the female brow is slightly higher, coursing above the orbital rim. The youthful female brow peaks at a point tangent to a line drawn from the nasal ala through the pupil or lateral limbus, and then tapers inferiorly (**Fig. 6**).

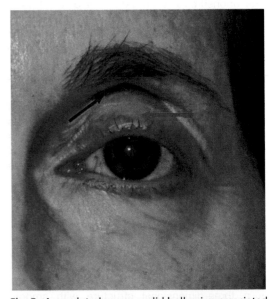

Fig. 5. Age-related upper eyelid hollowing associated with volume loss. Note the A-frame deformity (*black arrow*), and unmasked pretarsal eyelid associated with involution ptosis (*red arrow*). (*Courtesy of* Guy Massry, MD, Beverly Hills, CA.)

The youthful male brow is flatter and fuller, and runs over the orbital rim without the peak that is evident in women.[16]

Cutaneous changes also play a pivotal role in eyelid and periorbital aging. As skin ages, the dermal collagen matrix becomes fragmented and weakened, with impaired fibroblast function.[6] Instead of producing collagen and stabilizing the dermal matrix, damaged fibroblasts begin to create collagen-degrading enzymes, perpetuating the cycle. This degradation leads to the progressive loss of elasticity of the skin that, when paired with deflation, accentuates and deepens rhytids. In addition, laxity, pigmentary changes, and skin thinning occur.

MINIMALLY INVASIVE TREATMENT OF THE PERIORBITAL SKIN

Various surgical options exist for the correction of skin laxity. In the upper eyelid and brow, upper eyelid blepharoplasty and a variety of surgical brow lifting techniques are used to reduce skin redundancy and bulk. However, these modalities do nothing to improve skin quality and are inadequate for qualitatively improving skin appearance and texture.

Excellent skin care is the most important aspect of maintaining a youthful facial appearance. Tissue quality and skin reflectance depend on a consistent and ongoing commitment to such a regimen. All patients should use a basic facial moisturization

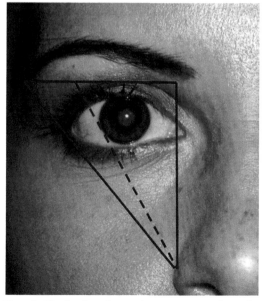

Fig. 6. Classic female eyebrow topography. The dotted line delineates the ideal peak of the brow arch. (*Courtesy of* Guy Massry, MD, Beverly Hills, CA.)

protocol as an integral part of their facial rejuvenation programs. This protocol should include direct application to the brows and upper lids. Daily sun protection with SPF (sun protection factor) 30 or greater is also integral to preventing the discoloration and degeneration of the upper eyelid and brow skin that results from ultraviolet light damage. Ultraviolet-blocking sunglasses and wide-brimmed hats are also important tools in preventing periocular photoaging.

Photoaging may be treated with several topical preparations, such as topical retinoids, hydroquinone, or alpha hydroxyl acids (AHAs).[30] Topical retinoids enhance hyaluronic acid deposition and increase the compaction of the stratum corneum, and topical AHAs increase epidermal thickness by enhancing synthesis of glycosaminoglycans, collagen, and elastic fibers.[30,31] Microdermabrasion and chemical peels, alone or in conjunction with retinoids, are also effective in reversing the signs of skin photoaging and in improving the appearance of scars and fine rhytids.[32] They deliver selective injury at a depth dictated by the technique used, enhancing collagen synthesis during the healing process. Superficial chemical peels using glycolic acid (20%–70%) or trichloroacetic acid (15%–35%) are a commonly used method of addressing fine lines in the eyelids.

Deeper peels with higher acid concentrations or the use of phenol may be associated with longer recovery, risk of hypopigmentation, and scarring. Any peel technique has a risk of causing reactivation of cutaneous herpetic infection, and a careful history and clinical evaluation must be performed. Some patients require pretreatment with antiviral agents before peeling procedures to mitigate this risk.[30] A comprehensive review of these treatments and techniques is beyond the scope of this article, but may be found in several recent reviews.[33–35]

Laser resurfacing has also gained popularity in recent decades as a reliable method of improving skin quality and reducing fine lines. In particular, CO_2 and erbium:ytrium aluminum garnet (Er:YAG) lasers are commonly used in the periorbital region for these purposes.[30,36] Lasers are able to target specific components of the skin, at specific depths to precisely deliver injury to the skin tissue.[37] CO_2 lasers, initially introduced in the 1980s, provide aggressive ablative therapy to the skin, but are associated with significant downtime. The laser emits light at a wavelength of 10,600 nm, which selectively targets water and vaporizes the epidermis as well as a variable thickness of dermis.[30,36] Fractionation of treatment decreases downtime and adverse effects. Overaggressive treatment with lasers may lead to adverse effects such as prolonged erythema, hyperpigmentation, milia, infections, hypersensitivity, scarring, and ectropion.[30] The Er:YAG laser emits energy in the infrared spectrum at 2940 nm, a wavelength that is also highly absorbed by water but is associated with less residual thermal damage.[30] Recovery is speedier with the Er:YAG versus the CO_2 laser, but the effect is also more subtle. Ablative therapy with the Er:YAG laser may also lead to the adverse effects listed earlier. Pigmentary anomalies are more likely in patients with dark skin.[15]

For mild laxity and rhytids, radiofrequency devices may also be used. Radiofrequency devices deliver thermal injury to the skin in several ways, including fractional bipolar devices, multi-source phase-controlled devices, monopolar devices, and combinations of these methods.[15] The thermal energy introduced by the devices does not ablate tissue, but focally injures it with subsequent tissue regeneration. Its effect is not altered by the type of pigmentation of the patient's skin. It has been shown to yield modest effects in reduction of rhytids.[15]

Microfocused ultrasonography (MFU) is another modality that may be used in mild cases of periorbital aging, without concern for pigmentation anomalies. Transducers generate ultrasonography energy of 4 to 7 MHz, which create zones of thermal microcoagulation 1 to 1.5 mm apart.[15] The energy may be delivered at a depth of 3 to 4.5 mm. Alam and colleagues[38] reported that the lateral brow may be elevated by applying MFU energy to the skin just above the lateral two-thirds of the eyebrow, with a mean elevation of 1.7 mm after treatment.

NEUROMODULATION

The United States Food and Drug Administration (FDA) has approved 3 injectable neuromodulators for aesthetic use, all derivatives of botulinum toxin. They function at the neuromuscular junction, cleaving proteins that are necessary for the release of acetylcholine from the axon's vesicles at the synapse.[1] The 3 approved toxins are abobotulinum toxin A (Dysport; Medicis, Scottsdale, AZ), incobotulinum toxin A (Xeomin; Merz Aesthetics, San Mateo, CA) and onabotulinum A (Botox; Allergan, Irvine, CA).[15] Xeomin is a so-called naked toxin, whereas the others are complexed to accessory proteins. The doses of Botox and Xeomin are roughly equivalent, whereas 2.5 units of Dysport are considered roughly equivalent to 1 unit of Botox or Xeomin.[15]

In the periorbita, neuromodulators can be used to efface hyperdynamic lines and to elevate, reshape, and improve the contour of the brow.

This article focuses on alterations of the brow, which are accomplished by selective reversible chemical denervation of opposing muscles that maintain brow height and position. As previously elaborated, the muscles that depress the brow are the orbital orbicularis oculi (lateral and medial brow) and the procerus and corrugators supercilii (medial brow).[19] Neuromodulation of the lateral orbital orbicularis reduces lateral brow depression (allows passive elevation), whereas similar treatment of the central brow depressors allows less opposed action of the frontalis, which results in an elevated central/medial brow. These selective denervation principals alter the native equilibrium of dynamic forces that act on the eyebrows allowing the desired changes. In general, the best candidates for this form of therapy are patients with better skin quality and less tissue laxity. Treatment of the frontalis muscle can be a useful manipulation on patients with high or arched brows, or those with poor lid closure such as can be seen after previous surgical alterations (**Figs. 7** and **8**). Care must be taken when manipulating the frontalis and periorbital musculature. Isolated selective relaxation of the medial frontalis (when treating medial brow depressors) sometimes yield an overly arched lateral brow, often called spocking of the brow (mephisto appearance).[1] This result occurs because the central frontalis muscle fibers are weakened relative to the lateral muscle fibers, allowing the lateral brow to disproportionately elevate and cause an unnatural arch (**Fig. 9**). In cases like these, staged relaxation of the lateral frontalis may be desired in order to reestablish a gentler upward sweep to the brow. Also, selective weakening of the glabellar muscles in isolation can splay the brows (increase interbrow distance) or cause unnatural elevation of the medial brow, altering the brow arch. In addition, eyelid ptosis can result from any periorbital injection. The authors' experience is that true eyelid ptosis (inferiorly displaced lid margin) results primarily from injections of the glabellar and lateral orbicularis muscles. In these cases the neurotoxin spreads to the eyelid. Pseudoptosis can also occur, typically from frontalis treatment, which can limit brow elevation or cause frank brow ptosis with secondary lid fullness. For these reasons, all manipulations with neurotoxin to the eyelids or periorbita require a proper evaluation, identification of patients at risk of complications, and sound judgment.

The technique for brow shaping with neuromodulators depends on the desired effect. For elevation of the lateral brow, the lateral orbicularis is selectively weakened. Four to 6 units of Xeomin or Botox (10–15 units of Dysport) are injected at

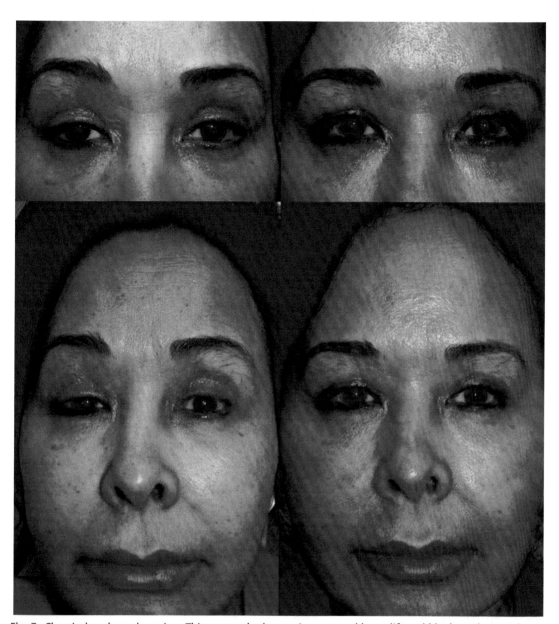

Fig. 7. Chemical eyebrow lowering. This woman had a previous coronal brow lift and blepharoplasty and complained of a surprised look, with arched brows and difficulty closing her eyes. (*Left*) Before and (*right*) after Botox treatment of the frontalis muscle to relax the forehead, lower the brows, and improve function and appearance. Above is frontal and below is full face views. (*Courtesy of* Guy Massry, MD, Beverly Hills, CA.)

1 or 2 points subdermally over the orbital orbicularis, in the area of maximum desired elevation (see **Fig. 8; Figs. 10** and **11**). The authors prefer subdermal injection because it tends to lead to less bruising with equally efficacious results as intramuscular injection.[39] In addition, in the delicate area of the brow (in close proximity to the eyelid) a more superficial injection may lead to less induced ptosis, which is always a potential concern. Also noteworthy is that needle gauge (G) can play a role in patient comfort. A recent

study has shown that when multiple areas are injected simultaneously, there is a statistically significant reduction in injection pain and increase in patient comfort when a 33-G versus 30-G needle is used. In addition bruising occurred less frequently with the 33-G needle, although this was not significant.[40]

For brow elevation, the optimal point for injection is identified visually and with palpation by asking the patient to frown aggressively and feeling for the maximum point of lateral brow

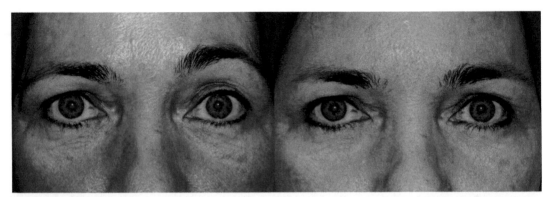

Fig. 8. This woman presented with native (nonoperated) asymmetric brows. The right temporal brow was elevated with selective neuromodulation of the lateral orbital orbicularis muscle, whereas the left brow was lowered with treatment of the frontalis muscle on that side. (*Courtesy of* Guy Massry, MD, Beverly Hills, CA.)

contraction. Ahn and colleagues[41] showed an average elevation in the central brow of 1 mm and of 4.8 mm in the lateral brow using this technique. In the author's experience, when lateral orbicularis treatment is augmented with injection of the upper crow's feet (upper lateral raphe) an increased lateral lift can be achieved. Although the authors have not evaluated this in a quantitative fashion, anecdotal observations have been positive. Medial brow elevation is achieved by targeting the procerus and corrugators supercilii muscles. Standard doses in this vary from 16 to 24 U of Botox and Xeomin and 40 to 60 U of Dysport. Treatment of the frontalis and brow depressors is often combined in such a way as to efface rhytids but still achieve desired changes in brow height or shape. This outcome is achieved by varying doses to specific muscle groups in a titrated fashion. It is important to identify patient needs when treating the medial brow complex.

Reducing hyperdynamic lines is generally straightforward, but, as stated, alterations in brow height, arch, and interbrow distance should be considered in the treatment protocol.

SOFT TISSUE FILLERS

As an appreciation of the role of volume loss and facial aging has emerged, so too has the application of soft tissue fillers in aesthetic facial rejuvenation. As such, soft tissue fillers have become one of the most important tools in the nonsurgical rejuvenation of the upper face.[42] There are 2 categories of soft tissue fillers: reversible or irreversible.[43,44] The authors prefer this distinction to temporary and permanent because reversibility is the key to avoiding permanent adverse events. The only class of reversible soft tissue fillers is the hyaluronic acid (HA) gels. HA exists naturally in the extracellular matrix of living organisms. The native molecule

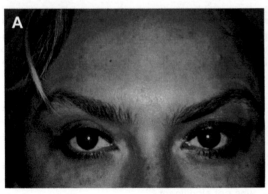
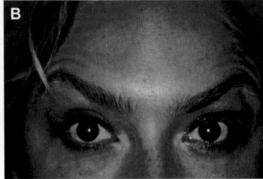

Fig. 9. Spock-like appearance after neuromodulation. When the corrugator muscles are treated superiorly, the frontalis muscle can also be affected, which allows lateral brow elevation relative to the central brow. (*A*) Without and (*B*) with forehead elevation. (*From* Yu CY, Nettar KD, Maas CS. Neuromodulators and fillers for periorbital rejuvenation. In: Massry GG, Murphy MR, Azizzadeh B, editors. Master techniques in blepharoplasty and periorbital rejuvenation. New York: Springer; 2011. p. 289–96; with permission.)

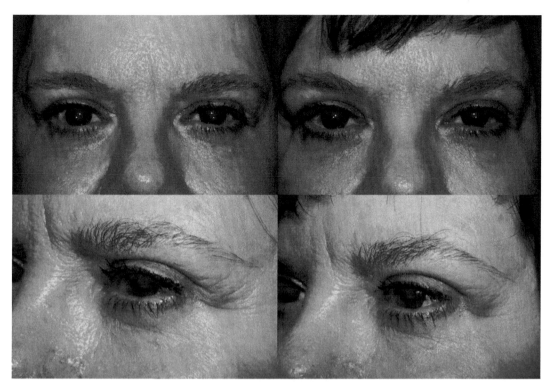

Fig. 10. Chemical brow lift. This woman is status post–upper blepharoplasty. She desired subtle lateral brow lift. (*Left above*) Frontal and (*left below*) oblique views before Botox® injection for temporal brow lift. (*Right*) After treatment. (*Courtesy of* Guy Massry, MD, Beverly Hills, CA.)

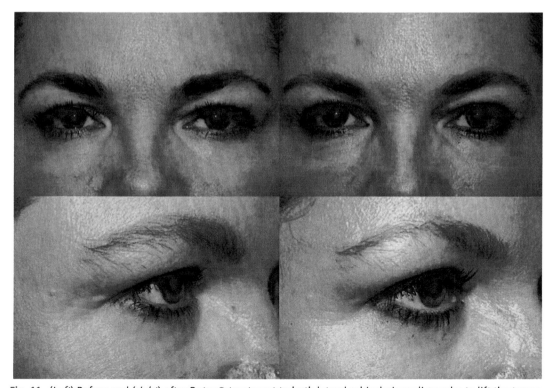

Fig. 11. (*Left*) Before and (*right*) after Botox® treatment to both lateral orbicularis oculi muscles to lift the temporal brow. Note improved brow arch on frontal (*above*) and oblique (*below*) views. (*Courtesy of* Guy Massry, MD, Beverly Hills, CA.)

has a short half-life of 1 to 2 days.[45–47] The process of cross-linking allows the creation of larger, longer lasting, and more stable gels.[42,48] The biochemical makeup of the various HA gels (degree of cross-linking and concentration) determines their individual properties and clinical effects, such as longevity, stability, hardness, and viscosity.[15,42] These characteristics guide clinical selection of an HA product for the desired effect.

Periorbital skin is thin and nonforgiving. For this reason, the authors consider this a high-risk area of treatment. Filling in this location must be approached with great care, knowledge of the various filler choices, and injection techniques to avoid adverse outcomes and patient dissatisfaction.[15,44] Inappropriate filler selection or injection technique can lead to fluid retention (hydrophilic reaction), contour irregularities, and an unnatural bluish color change to the skin (Tyndall effect).[44,48] Hydrophilic reactions are a result of higher concentration HA gel (greater osmotic effect), which is often placed too superficially. In the author's experience this has more commonly been seen with the Juvéderm family of products (concentration, 24 mg/mL) compared with Restylane (20 mg/mL), and least commonly with the use of Belotero. Contour irregularities occur from too much or too superficial placement of product. They can also be associated with an inflammatory reaction to the product. The Tyndall effect is simply light scattering from particles in a suspension (Fig. 12).[42] These issues are much more prevalent around the eyes in lower lid treatment, because the lid/cheek interface depression (tear trough, orbitomalar groove) in that location underlie thinner skin than that of the brow and brow/upper lid transition. Because HA products are reversible they are especially useful in treatment to the higher risk locations of eyelids and surrounding areas.

Hyaluronidase (HYAL) is an enzyme that degrades HA and reverses its effect.[42,44,49] There are a variety of different HYAL products available, with the clinical selection of HYAL product dependent on preference of the injector.[49] Because HYAL allows rapid degradation of HA it should always be available when injecting anywhere on the face.[44]

The HA fillers that are FDA approved in the United States for aesthetic purposes are in 4 families based on how they are manufactured and their biochemical makeup: (1) nonanimal stabilized HA (NASHA) products (Restylane and Perlane [Medicis]), (2) Hylacross™ products (Juvéderm Ultra, Ultra Plus, and Voluma [Allergan]), (3) cohesive polydensified matrix (CPM) HA (Belotero Balance [Merz]), and (4) products with low HA concentration (Prevelle Silk [Mentor]).[15,42] The first 3 families all have HA concentrations between 20 and 24 mg/mL and Prevelle has a concentration of 5.5 mg/mL. The higher the filler concentration the greater the tendency to bind water. In the periorbital area the authors prefer Restylane and Belotero, based on their rheologic characteristics. The specific rheology of each product imparts a particular individualized clinical effect.[50,51] The 2 flow (rheologic) parameters of importance are the G′ (elastic modulus) and viscosity of the particular gel. The G′ is the stiffness of the gel. High-G′ gels are stiffer and contribute to tissue vectoring (lifting) and resistance to deformation from the forces of gravity and facial movement. The viscosity of a gel is the ability to resist tissue spread and stay in place, thus contributing to contour stability. Restylane (NASHA product) has both a high G′ and high viscosity. Thus it imparts a powerful and stable lift and fill and is best implanted deep (subdermally) for maximum effect. Belotero (CPM product) has the opposite rheologic properties, with both a low G′ and low viscosity. This product spreads

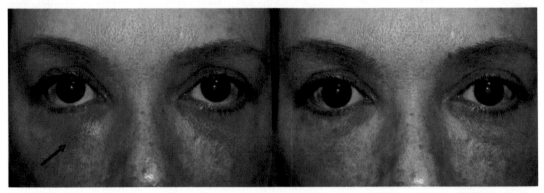

Fig. 12. (*Left*) Bluish discoloration (Tyndall reaction) and hydrophilic response in the right lower lid from previous Juvederm injection (*arrow*). Reduction of both after hyaluronidase injection (*right*). (*Courtesy of* Guy Massry, MD, Beverly Hills, CA.)

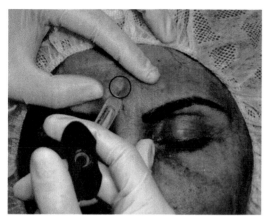

Fig. 13. Superficial injection of Belotero to glabellar rhytids. Blanching in this instance is a normal finding. (*Courtesy of* Hema Sundarem, MD, Rockville, MD.)

within tissue and has less tendency to lift compared with Restylane. For this reason Belotero is better suited for superficial placement. Belotero also has the least tendency for Tyndall reaction because it lacks a prominent particulate phase.[42] The Juvéderm family of products has the highest concentration and, as stated, the authors do not use them in the eyelids or adjacent areas because they tend to produce a higher incidence of hydrophilic reaction and Tyndall effect. By virtue of their concentration and high cross link percentage they are also the most difficult products to remove with HYAL. These HA gel characteristics are essential to understanding product selection and depth of placement in the periocular area.

As a result of its flow characteristics Belotero may be injected intradermally to efface fine lines.[52] Previous to this application, fine-line treatment was only safely accomplished with HA gel which was diluted (Juvéderm) to make the product more user friendly and complication free for this purpose.[53] Intradermal (superficial) Belotero

injection requires a serial puncture or threading technique with a fine needle until slight blanching of the skin is seen. This technique is useful for effacing glabellar lines (**Fig. 13**). In this instance, blanching is a normal consequence of filler treatment as blood vessels are displaced. However, with deeper subdermal injections for volumetric enhancement, blanching is an ominous sign suggesting potential ischemic reaction.

The author's technique for filling and lifting the brows involves deep implantation of Restylane to the lateral two-thirds of the brow. The filler may be injected using a serial puncture technique with a sharp needle, or with a blunt cannula fanning from a single skin puncture site. The authors prefer the use of a blunt cannula because they think it leads to less bruising and may reduce the incidence of vascular occlusion (**Fig. 14**).[54,55] The ideal plane for filler placement is subgaleal or preperiosteal. The filler may also be placed into the area of the inferior brow fat pad or superior sulcus to camouflage eyelid hollows (**Fig. 15**). Filling this hollow restores the reflective contour of the upper lid and reduces the intervening shadows that are typical of aging or previous surgery. Temporal wasting is another age-related change often seen in thin women. Restylane and Juvéderm injected subdermally may enhance youthfulness by effacing these temporal hollows.[6]

Besides the complications mentioned previously (hydrophilic reaction, contour issues, and Tyndall effect), more serious adverse events can occur with soft tissue filler injections. These events include infection, biofilm reaction, cutaneous vascular compromise (skin/tissue necrosis); and, most worrisome, blindness from retrograde injection into the ocular arterial system. The scope of this discussion and management of these issues is long and detailed and is reviewed in detail by DeLorenzi.[44,56]

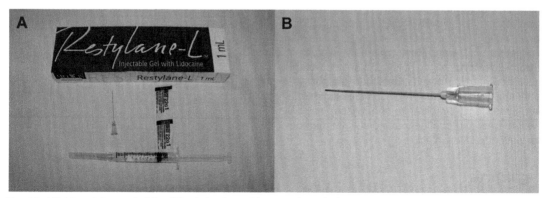

Fig. 14. (*A*) Materials needed for filler injection with cannula include HA gel, local anesthetic, 22-G needle to create entry point, and (*B*) cannula. (*Courtesy of* Guy Massry, MD, Beverly Hills, CA.)

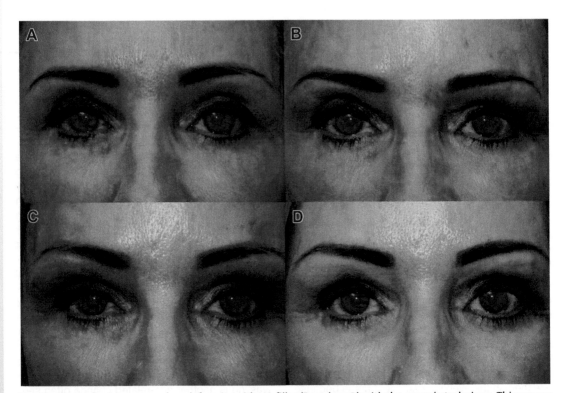

Fig. 15. Camouflaging upper sulcus deformity with HA filler (Restylane®) with the cannula technique. This woman presented with severe hollowing after upper blepharoplasty. (*A*) Prior to treatment with Restylane, (*B*) immediate result after filling left upper lid, (*C*) right upper lid, and (*D*) final result at 6 weeks. The filler was primarily applied to the brow fat pad and superior orbit. (*Courtesy of* Guy Massry, MD, Beverly Hills, CA.)

SUMMARY

Minimally or less-invasive procedures for facial rejuvenation have increased in total number, in percentage of all aesthetic procedures performed, in market share, and in overall revenue generated over the last decade.[57] This increase has been driven by a reduction in procedural risk, recovery, and cost. As such, to stay current and provide a complete array of treatment options to patients, it is incumbent on facial surgeons to become familiar and comfortable with the varied nonsurgical interventions reviewed in this article, particularly relating to the delicate and high-risk eyelid and periorbital area. Most assuredly over time, there will be limits to the utility of these non-surgical interventions. However, until then, the ability to offer these less invasive enhancements to patients in a consistently predictable and reliable way will nurture trust and confidence and solidify the doctor/patient relationship.

REFERENCES

1. Yu CY, Nettar KD, Mass CS. Neuromodulators and fillers for periorbital rejuvenation. In: Massry GG, Murphy M, Azizzadeh B, editors. Master techniques in blepharoplasty and periorbital rejuvenation. New York: Springer; 2011. p. 259–72.
2. Carruthers J, Glogau RG, Blitzer A, et al. Advances in facial rejuvenation: botulinum toxin type a, hyaluronic acid dermal fillers, and combination therapies—consensus recommendations. Plast Reconstr Surg 2008;121(Suppl 5):5S–29S.
3. Lambros VS. The dynamics of facial aging. Paper presented at the Annual Meeting of the American Society for Aesthetic Plastic Surgery. Las Vegas (NV). April 27–May 3, 2002.
4. Donath AS, Glasgold R, Glasgold M. Volume loss versus gravity: new concepts in facial aging. Curr Opin Otolaryngol Head Neck Surg 2007;15(4):238–43.
5. Lambros V. Observations on periorbital and midface aging. Plast Reconstr Surg 2007;120(5):1367–76 [discussion: 1377].
6. Fitzgerald R. Contemporary concepts in brow and eyelid aging. Clin Plast Surg 2013;40:21–42.
7. Lam S, Glasgold M, Glasgold R. Complementary fat grafting. Philadelphia: Lippincott Williams & Wilkins; 2007.
8. Glassgold RA, Lam SM, Glassgold MJ. Periorbital fat grafting. In: Massry GG, Murphy M, Azizzadeh B, editors. Master techniques in blepharoplasty and

periorbital rejuvenation. New York: Springer; 2011. p. 259–72.

9. Massry G, Hartstein M. The lift and fill lower blepharoplasty. Ophthal Plast Reconstr Surg 2012;28(3): 213–8.

10. Massry GG. Commentary on "The sigmoidal upper blepharoplasty". Ophthal Plast Reconstr Surg 2012;28:454.

11. Massry GG. Comprehensive lower eyelid rejuvenation. Facial Plast Surg 2010;26:209–21.

12. Massry GG, Azizzadeh B. Periorbital fat grafting. Facial Plast Surg 2013;29:46–57.

13. American Society for Aesthetic Plastic Surgery. 2011 Cosmetic surgery national data bank: 2011 statistics. Available at: http://www.surgery.org/download/2011stats.pdf. Accessed March 10, 2012.

14. Smith L, Cockerham K. Hyaluronic acid dermal fillers: can adjunctive lidocaine improve patient satisfaction without decreasing efficacy or duration? Patient Prefer Adherence 2011;5:133–9.

15. Sundaram H, Kiripolsky M. Nonsurgical rejuvenation of the upper eyelid and brow. Clin Plast Surg 2013; 40:55–76.

16. Massry G. The external browpexy. Ophthal Plast Reconstr Surg 2012;28(2):90–5.

17. Czyz CN, Hill RH, Foster JA. Preoperative evaluation of the brow-lid continuum. Clin Plast Surg 2013;40: 43–53.

18. Georgescu D, Belsare G, McCann JD, et al. Adjunctive procedures in upper eyelid blepharoplasty: internal brow fat sculpting and elevation, glabellar myectomy, and lacrimal gland repositioning. In: Massry GG, Murphy MR, Azizzadeh B, editors. Master techniques in blepharoplasty and periorbital rejuvenation. New York: Springer; 2011. p. 101–8.

19. Tan KS, Oh SR, Priel A, et al. Surgical anatomy of the forehead eyelids and midface for the aesthetic surgeon. In: Massry GG, Murphy MR, Azizzadeh B, editors. Master techniques in blepharoplasty and periorbital rejuvenation. New York: Springer; 2011. p. 11–24.

20. Putterman AM, Urist MJ. Surgical anatomy of the orbital septum. Ann Ophthalmol 1974;6:290–4.

21. Meyer DR, Linberg JV, Wobig JL. Anatomy of the orbital septum and associated eyelid connective tissues. Implications for ptosis surgery. Ophthal Plast Reconstr Surg 1991;7:104–13.

22. Seiff SR, Seiff BD. Anatomy of the Asian eyelid. Facial Plast Surg Clin North Am 2007;15:309–14.

23. Massry G. Nasal fat preservation in upper eyelid blepharoplasty. Ophthal Plast Reconstr Surg 2011; 27:352–5.

24. Yoo DB, Peng G, Massry GG. Effacing the orbitoglabellar groove with transposed upper eyelid fat. Ophthal Plast Reconstr Surg 2013;29:220–4.

25. Morton AD. Upper eyelid blepharoplasty. In: Massry GG, Murphy MR, Azizzadeh B, editors.

Master techniques in blepharoplasty and periorbital rejuvenation. New York: Springer; 2011. p. 87–99.

26. Matros E, Garcia JA, Yaremchuk MJ. Change in eyebrow position and shape with ageing. Plast Reconstr Surg 2009;124:1296–301.

27. Patil SB, Kale SM, Jaiswal S, et al. Effect of aging on the shape and position of the eyebrow in an Indian population. Aesthetic Plast Surg 2011;35:1031–5.

28. Buchanan A, Holds JB. The beautiful eye: perception of beauty in the periocular area. In: Massry GG, Murphy MR, Azizzadeh B, editors. Master techniques in blepharoplasty and periorbital rejuvenation. New York: Springer; 2011. p. 25–9.

29. Pessa JE, Chen Y. Curve analysis of the aging orbital aperture. Plast Reconstr Surg 2002;109:751.

30. Manaloto RM, Alster TS. Periorbital rejuvenation: a review of dermatologic treatments. Dermatol Surg 1999;25(1):1–9.

31. Ditre CM, Griffin TD, Murphy GF, et al. Effects of alpha-hydroxy acids on photoaged skin: a pilot clinical, histologic, and ultrastructural study. J Am Acad Dermatol 1996;34(2 Pt 1):187–95.

32. Hubbard BA, Unger JG, Rohrich RJ. Reversal of skin aging with topical retinoids. Plast Reconstr Surg 2014;133(4):481e–90e.

33. Brody HJ, Monheit GD, Resnik SS, et al. A history of chemical peeling. Dermatol Surg 2000;26(5):405–9.

34. Taylor SC, Badreshia-Bansal S, Callender VD, et al. Chemical peels. In: Treatments for skin of color. Philadelphia: Saunders; 2011. p. 315–20.

35. Jackson A. Chemical peels. Facial Plast Surg 2014; 30:26–34.

36. Ross EV, Miller C, Meehan K, et al. One-pass CO2 versus multiple-pass Er:YAG laser resurfacing in the treatment of rhytides: a comparison side-by-side study of pulsed CO2 and Er:YAG lasers. Dermatol Surg 2001;27(8):709–15. Available at: http://www.ncbi.nlm.nih.gov/pubmed/11493293.

37. Brauer JA, Patel U, Hale EK. Laser skin resurfacing, chemical peels, and other cutaneous treatments of the brow and upper lid. Clin Plast Surg 2013; 40(1):91–9.

38. Alam M, White LE, Martin N, et al. Ultrasound tightening of facial and neck skin: a rater blinded prospective cohort study. J Am Acad Dermatol 2010; 62:262–9.

39. Gordin EA, Luginbuhl AL, Ortlip T, et al. Subcutaneous vs intramuscular botulinum toxin split-face randomized study. JAMA Facial Plast Surg 2014;16: 193–8.

40. Sezgin B, Ozel B, Bulam H, et al. The effect of microneedle thickness on pain during minimally invasive facial procedures: a clinical study. Aesthet Surg J 2014;34:757–65.

41. Ahn MS, Catten M, Maas CS. Temporal brow lift using botulinum toxin A. Plast Reconstr Surg 2000; 105(3):1129–35 [discussion: 1136–9].

42. Sundaram H, Cassuto D. Biophysical characteristics of hyaluronic acid soft-tissue fillers and their relevance to aesthetic applications. Plast Reconstr Surg 2013;132:5S–21S.

43. Smith KC. Reversible vs nonreversible fillers in facial aesthetics: concerns and considerations. Dermatol Online J 2008;14:3.

44. DeLorenzi C. Complications of injectable fillers, part I. Aesthet Surg J 2013;33:561–75.

45. Laurent TC. Biochemistry of hyaluronan. Acta Otolaryngol Suppl 1987;442:7–24.

46. Laurent TC, Dahl IM, Dahl LB, et al. The catabolic fate of hyaluronic acid. Connect Tissue Res 1986; 15:33–41.

47. Fraser JR, Laurent TC, Engstrom-Laurent A, et al. Elimination of hyaluronic acid from the blood stream in the human. Clin Exp Pharmacol Physiol 1984;11:17–25.

48. Kontis TC. Contemporary review of injectable facial fillers. JAMA Facial Plast Surg 2013;15:58–64.

49. Cavallini M, Gazzola R, Metalla M, et al. The role of hyaluronidase in the treatment of complications from hyaluronic acid dermal fillers. Aesthet Surg J 2013;33:1167–74.

50. Sundaram H, Voigts B, Beer K, et al. Comparison of the rheological properties of viscosity and elasticity in two categories of soft tissue fillers: calcium hydroxylapatite and hyaluronic acid. Dermatol Surg 2010;36(Suppl 3):1859S–65S.

51. Stocks D, Sundaram H, Michaels J, et al. Rheological evaluation of the physical properties of hyaluronic acid dermal fillers. J Drugs Dermatol 2011;10(9): 974–80.

52. Micheels P, Sarazin D, Besse S, et al. A blanching technique for intradermal injection of the hyaluronic acid Belotero. Plast Reconstr Surg 2013;132: 59S–68S.

53. Fagien S, Cassuto D. Reconstituted injectable hyaluronic acid: expanded applications in facial aesthetics and additional thoughts on the mechanism of action in cosmetic medicine. Plast Reconstr Surg 2012;130:208–17.

54. Zeichner JA, Cohen JL. Use of blunt tipped cannulas for soft tissue fillers. J Drugs Dermatol 2012; 11(1):70–2.

55. Cassuto D. Blunt-tipped microcannulas for filler injection: an ethical duty? J Drugs Dermatol 2012; 11(8):s42.

56. DeLorenzi C. Complications of injectable fillers, part 2: vascular complications. Aesthet Surg J 2014;34: 584–600.

57. Wilson S, Soares M, Reavey P, et al. Trends and drivers of the aesthetic market during a turbulent economy. Plast Reconstr Surg 2014;133:783e–9e.

Surgical Treatment of the Brow and Upper Eyelid

Scott Shadfar, MD[a],*, Stephen W. Perkins, MD[a,b]

KEYWORDS

- Blepharoplasty • Upper eyelid • Forehead lift • Brow lift • Upper facial rejuvenation

KEY POINTS

- The surgeon must be meticulous when marking the patient for upper eyelid blepharoplasty before surgery, and the surgeon should make use of a fine-tip marker and small calipers.
- The age-related changes in the eyelid and eyebrow continuum are multifactorial, with volume loss or deflation (bony and fat atrophy) taking on an equivalent contribution in the aging process as the classically described tissue descent and skin changes.
- The frontal hairline, slope of the forehead, and structure of the underlying frontal bone should be considered when preparing for and choosing any surgical intervention to ensure proper approach selection and incision placement.
- The key to guiding and stabilizing brow position is releasing the periosteum at the arcus marginalis.
- Patients with hairlines that prevent a standard endoscopic approach may benefit from a combination procedure using trichophytic or transverse mid-forehead incisions to address medial brow ptosis.

INTRODUCTION

The periorbital region and upper third of the face are often the first facial areas to show signs of aging, with patients presenting with subjective complaints of having an unrested, angry, or sad appearance. Upper facial aging commonly manifests as brow ptosis, upper facial dynamic and static rhytids, volume loss and periorbital hollowing, with associated prolapse of periorbital fat, and dermatochalasis.[1,2]

The brow and upper lid anatomy, as well as the aging and esthetic analysis, are described in further detail within the earlier portions of this issue. When evaluating a patient for surgical intervention, the relationship of the upper eyelids relative to the other structures forming the upper third of the face, including the eyelid margin position, eyebrows, forehead, and the location of the frontal hairline should be analyzed in continuity.[3]

The expression, brow-eyelid continuum, has been accepted by surgeons, and can be used to counsel patients and draw attention to the fact that treatment of these structures relative to each other, as opposed to in isolation, will allow the surgeon to achieve a more harmonious and esthetically pleasing rejuvenation.[3]

The age-related changes in the eyelid and eyebrow continuum are multifactorial, similar to other regions of the face. Several philosophies describe aging as a 3-dimensional process, with volume loss, deflation, and bony and fat atrophy taking on an equivalent contribution in the aging process, as the classically described tissue descent and skin changes. These changes include the rhytids, skin thinning, and laxity seen with loss of dermal collagen and solar damage.[1,4–6]

The surgeon must carefully assess each factor individually and recognize the interrelationship between the characteristic aging patterns and the

Disclosures: The authors have no financial disclosures.
[a] Meridian Plastic Surgeons, 170 West 106th Street, Indianapolis, IN 46290, USA; [b] Department of Otolaryngology/Head and Neck Surgery, Indiana University School of Medicine, 705 Riley Hospital Drive, RI0860, Indianapolis, IN 46202-5230, USA
* Corresponding author. 170 West 106th Street, Indianapolis, IN 46290.
E-mail addresses: DrShadfar@gmail.com; Sperkski@gmail.com

facialplastic.theclinics.com

surrounding anatomic structures to select the appropriate treatment. In this article, the authors explore the various approaches and techniques available for surgical rejuvenation of the upper face, including the upper periorbital region.

PREOPERATIVE PLANNING AND PREPARATION

The optimal results begin with appropriate preoperative planning and preparation. The surgeon should have a clear understanding of the surgical and nonsurgical techniques available to achieve the desired outcome and meet the expectations of the patient and surgeon alike. Considerations into the etiology of each patient's complaints and anatomic findings should be weighed against the effect that the procedure will have on the brow-lid continuum. This will allow the surgeon to accomplish the shared goals, while avoiding or reducing the need for revisions or further corrective procedures.[1]

Assessment of the patient's brow should include the brow position, height, brow curvature or arch, and the brow's relationship to the upper eyelids and hairline. The surgical techniques in brow elevation or stabilization aim to reshape the brow position relative to the adjacent forehead and upper eyelid skin. The surgeon should be conscientious that an overly elevated brow may not only result in a surprised look but also impart an aged appearance.[7,8]

The frontal hairline, slope of the forehead, and structure of the underlying frontal bone should be considered as well when choosing the appropriate surgical approach and incision placement (**Table 1**).[9,10] Additionally, documenting hyperfunctional brow musculature (corrugator supercilii, procerus, frontalis, orbicularis) may persuade the surgeon to consider myotomies or myectomies during their surgical intervention to reduce skin wrinkling.[7,11,12]

Blepharoplasty of the upper eyelid is indicated when the eyelids require contouring due to excessive or redundant upper eyelid skin, or when herniated periorbital fat calls for resection and redistribution. The preoperative evaluation should include critical evaluation of the skin, orbicularis muscle, prolapsed fat, the size and position of the lacrimal gland, levator palpebrae superioris function, and the position of the upper eyelid relative to the pupillary light reflex.[1] The limitations of blepharoplasty and the role of adjuvant procedures must be discussed with the patient. Nonsurgical management using botulinum toxin would be a more suitable treatment for the patient with significant crow's feet requesting periorbital rejuvenation. Similarly, the patient with fine wrinkling and "crepe paper" skin may achieve significant improvement with skin resurfacing, as opposed to blepharoplasty.[7] For those patients with volume loss contributing to the signs of periorbital aging, volumizing the brow with hyaluronic acid fillers or autologous fat may help give a more youthful appearance to the brow and periorbital region.[2,13,14]

The preoperative assessment of the patient seeking rejuvenation of the brow and upper eyelid complex should include a complete medical history to evaluate for systemic disease processes, such as autoimmune or collagen vascular diseases, endocrinopathies with ocular manifestations, dry eye symptoms, and visual acuity changes.[7] Often ocular physical examination findings can be a manifestation of a systemic disease process, such as allergy or thyroid-associated exophthalmos, and it is important to distinguish whether the changes to the brow and upper eyelids are truly related to hereditary or age-related changes (dermatochalasis and steatoblepharon). Comorbidities may have ocular consequences as well, and the appropriate workup should be completed, including blood levels of thyroid-stimulating hormone if thyroid-related endocrinopathies are suspected, in addition to consultation with an endocrinologist or ophthalmologist when indicated. Any patient with history of dry eye or visual acuity changes should be evaluated by an ophthalmologist.[7]

UPPER EYELID REJUVENATION
Patient Marking and Positioning

The surgeon must be meticulous when marking the patient for upper eyelid blepharoplasty before surgery, and the surgeon should make use of a fine-tip marker and small calipers. The patient may be marked in a seated or supine position, as long as the surgeon accounts for the tissues of the brow being drawn artificially higher in a supine position compared with when the patient is seated.

A difference of 1 to 3 mm from one eyelid to the next may create perceptible asymmetries. The surgeon's contralateral hand is used to reposition or brace the eyebrow superiorly, isolating the perceived contribution of brow ptosis from true upper eyelid dermatochalasis. Alternatively, if a forehead lift is indicated at the same time as the upper eyelid blepharoplasty, the surgeon may elect to perform the forehead lift first, and then measure and mark the appropriate amount of upper eyelid skin excision necessary to provide rejuvenation of the upper eyelid complex, so as to minimize the risk of lagophthalmos.[7]

Table 1
Approaches for corrective surgery of the brow and forehead

Type of Lift	Incision	Dissection	Suspension	Selection	Advantages	Disadvantages
Coronal	Parallels frontal hairline (5–7 cm back)	Subgaleal	No	Classic operation for most women unless they have a high frontal hairline, not good for male patients	Incision hidden in hairline, good exposure to forehead muscles	Elevation of frontal hairline, scalp anesthesia behind incision
Endoscopic	Paramedian 2 cm posterior to hairline, and lateral aligned with lateral canthus	Subperiosteal	Suspend using bone tunnel or fixation device	Best operation for men or women, unless they have a high frontal hairline, may use combination approach	Incisions hidden in hairline, good exposure to forehead muscles, shorter operative time, minimal closure time	Elevation of frontal hairline, scalp anesthesia, necessitates specialized equipment
Pretrichial or trichophytic	Beveled posterior to anterior, incision just at or anterior to frontal hairline	Subgaleal or subperiosteal	No	Good option for women with thick hair, high frontal hairline, may be combined with endoscopic approach for patients with high hairlines	Does not raise hairline, direct access to forehead muscles, good scar camouflage is possible	Scalp anesthesia behind incision, technically more difficult, scar may be visible if not executed correctly
Combination mid-forehead transverse incision with endoscopic approach	Midline forehead crease, between neurovascular bundles; standard lateral endoscopic incisions	Subperiosteal	Laterally similar to endoscopic approach	Good option for men with prominent forehead rhytids, and significant male pattern baldness or shaved head	Direct access to forehead muscles, good scar camouflage is possible	Incision may leave obvious scar in area not easily camouflaged
Traditional mid-brow	Hidden in forehead creases, not a straight line	Subcutaneous	Suspend upper orbicularis muscle to periosteum at upper skin margin	Good when scar can be hidden in deep forehead crease, or patients with male pattern baldness	Selective skin excision, precise brow elevation	Incision may leave obvious scar in area not easily camouflaged
Direct	Skin excision in forehead crease just above eyebrow	Subcutaneous	Suspend transverse orbicularis muscle to subgaleal tissue above brow	Elderly patient with deep furrows over the brows, functional elevation of brow, unilateral brow ptosis	Precise brow elevation, minimal edema or ecchymosis	Incision is difficult to camouflage, no change in mimetic function so brow may descend with time, can distort existing forehead furrows

Adapted from Chand M, Perkins SW. Comparison of surgical approaches for upper facial rejuvenation. Curr Opin Otolaryngol Head Neck Surg 2000;8(4):326–31; with permission.

The marking begins with the patient looking up, and the supratarsal crease is identified and measured from the eyelid margin using small calipers; this denotes the location of the inferior limb of the surgical marking. This measurement ranges from 8 to 10 mm from the lid margin (8–10 mm in women; 8–9 mm in men) (**Fig. 1**).

The inferior limb of the marking is curved gently and parallels the lid margin; the inferior limb of the marking is carried medially to within 1 to 2 mm of the punctum and laterally to the lateral canthus. Medially, the nasal-orbital depression should not be violated, as an incision in this area may result in a webbed scar; ending the incision medially within 1 to 2 mm of the punctum avoids this result. If the marking is carried along the curve of the eyelid crease lateral to the lateral canthus, the final closure scar line will bring the upper eyelid tissue downward, thus resulting in a hooded appearance. In an effort to avoid this unsightly result, the marking sweeps diagonally *upward* from the lateral canthus to the lateral eyebrow margin (**Fig. 2**). This modification of the lateral incision resists lateral hooding and can be easily camouflaged with makeup.

Next, the superior limb of the surgical marking is made. This is facilitated by using smooth forceps to pinch the excess amount of upper eyelid skin so that the lashes roll upward (**Fig. 3**). This conservative maneuver avoids over-resection of upper lid skin and reduces the risk of lagophthalmos as a long-term complication.

The authors elect to sit while performing brow and eyelid surgery. The patient is placed in a supine position with the surgeon on the side of the eye to be addressed and the assistant is seated across. Stabilization of the skin in the eyelid is

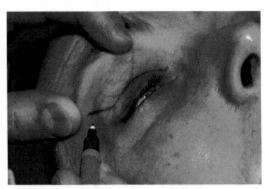

Fig. 2. The marking sweeps diagonally upward from the lateral canthus to the lateral eyebrow margin to avoid a hooded appearance with closure.

paramount to making the skin-only incision of the upper eyelid; therefore, it is the assistant's role to place tension on the skin. At the time of the brow lift, the surgeon and assistant should position themselves at the head of the bed (**Fig. 4**).

Surgical Technique for the Upper Eyelid

Generally, isolated upper eyelid blepharoplasty can be performed under local anesthesia with or

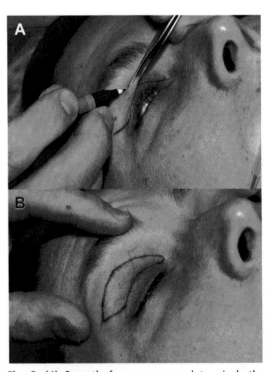

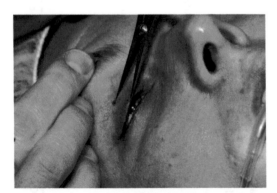

Fig. 1. The supratarsal crease is identified with the patient looking upward; the supratarsal crease is then measured from the lid margin using small calipers. This measurement denotes the location of the inferior limb of the surgical marking and varies based on sex of the patient.

Fig. 3. (*A*) Smooth forceps are used to pinch the excess amount of upper eyelid skin to roll the eyelashes upward denoting the superior limb of the surgical marking. (*B*) The superior limb is connected with the inferior limb medially and laterally with sweeping diagonal marks.

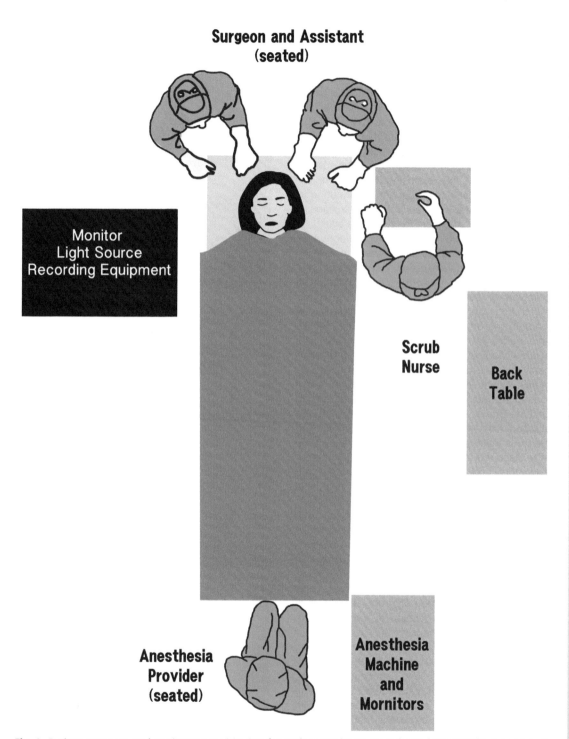

Fig. 4. Patient, surgeon, and equipment positioning for endoscopic brow procedures. (*Adapted from* Javidnia H, Sykes J. Endoscopic brow lifts: have they replaced coronal lifts? Facial Plast Surg Clin North Am 2013;21(2):195; with permission.)

without intravenous sedation for patient comfort, or a general anesthetic may be instituted during concomitant rejuvenative procedures, including forehead or brow lift. Lidocaine 2% with epinephrine (1:50,000) is infiltrated deep to the skin but superficial to the orbicularis oculi muscle, thus minimizing the risk of ecchymosis caused by the injection of local anesthesia.

A round-handled scalpel with a #15 Bard-Parker blade is ideal for following the curves of the surgical markings in the upper eyelid. Once the skin incision is made, the skin is then sharply dissected from the underlying orbicularis oculi muscle with a scalpel blade or dissecting beveled scissors. The preseptal orbicularis oculi muscle is then evaluated. If it is atrophic or very thin, then the muscle need not be excised; however, most often, a thin strip of preseptal orbicularis oculi muscle is excised medially, thus exposing the fat compartments. If the muscle is robust and contributing to the aged appearance, then a narrow excision is performed along the entire length of the eyelid.

Attention is then directed to the pseudoherniation of orbital fat. If there is fullness of the upper eyelid, a conservative excision, if any, can be performed, with care to avoid the late sequela of the hollowed or sunken appearance to the upper eyelid from over-resection. A small opening is made in the orbital septum overlying the middle and medial fat compartments. Attentiveness is needed to avoid the intervening trochlea and superior oblique muscle separating these compartments. Gentle pressure on the globe can reveal redundant fat from each compartment. Using Griffiths-Brown forceps, the herniated fat is grasped from its respective compartment, and the fat is infiltrated with local anesthesia to minimize discomfort associated with subsequent electrocautery and excision of the redundant fat, unless the patient is under general anesthesia (**Fig. 5**). Meticulous hemostasis is of utmost importance, not only to maintain a clear operative field, but also to minimize the risk of postoperative bleeding. Once fat removal from both compartments is completed, bipolar electrocautery is used to ensure hemostasis before wound closure.

The preferred technique for skin closure is as follows (**Fig. 6**): 7–0 blue polypropylene suture is used in an interrupted fashion to reapproximate the skin edges. Previously, the senior author (S.W.P.) used 6–0 mild chromic or fast-absorbing gut sutures; however, patients often developed inflammatory responses and subsequent milia, which have rarely been encountered since using interrupted 7–0 sized suture. The upper eyelid blepharoplasty incision closure is then reinforced with a running 6–0 blue polypropylene suture in a subcuticular fashion, with knots tied at the medial and lateral aspects of the incision.

FOREHEAD AND BROW REJUVENATION
Patient Marking and Positioning

Although the nonendoscopic approaches (coronal or trichophytic) have been the standard by with

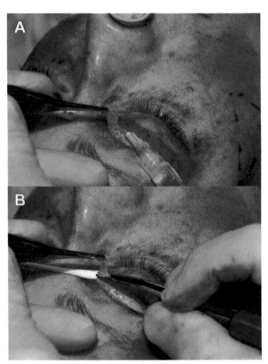

Fig. 5. A small opening is made in the orbital septum to access the middle and medial fat compartments. Gentle pressure on the globe demonstrates redundant fat from each compartment. (*A*) Forceps are used to grasp the herniated fat and local anesthesia is infiltrated at the base of the herniated fat. (*B*) Conservative excision of the fat is then performed once the base is cauterized.

which all other techniques have been compared, there has been a trend toward, and wider acceptance of, the endoscopic brow lift, which is our preferred method for surgical rejuvenation of the

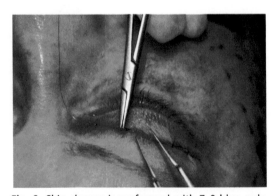

Fig. 6. Skin closure is performed with 7–0 blue polypropylene sutures used in an interrupted fashion to reapproximate the skin edges; the remainder of the skin closure is performed with 6–0 blue polypropylene suture in a subcuticular fashion with knots tied at the medial and lateral ends.

brow. Summaries of the standard approaches are outlined in **Table 1**.

The standard endoscopic brow technique in all cases places bilateral incisions laterally, 2 cm posterior to the temporal hairline recession at a location demarcated by the lateral canthus and temporal line. Additionally, 2 paramedian incisions are made to gain access medially. In the preoperative holding area, the surgical markings are made and the patient's hair is twirled (**Fig. 7**). Patients with a large slope or curvature to the forehead, or patients with high hairlines, can still benefit from an endoscopic approach using a midline modified trichophytic incision, in addition to the standard laterally positioned incisions (**Fig. 8**).

Previous limitations to the endoscopic approach included treating those patients with high hairlines or large foreheads, prominent male pattern baldness, or patients with shaved heads. Using a modified combination approach with a midline transverse forehead incision and the standard endoscopic temporal incisions, this patient population can benefit from endoscopic brow lift with inconspicuous scars (**Fig. 9**). Generally, these incisions are planned in prominent forehead creases to aid in camouflaging the scars.

Surgical Technique for the Forehead/Brow

Many techniques for surgical rejuvenation of the upper third of the face have been described in the literature. Coronal forehead lifts are no longer used in our practice, and this article focuses on our standard endoscopic approach with modifications in the technique for special clinical scenarios, broadening the indications for the endoscopic approach.

Before incisions or local infiltration, historically the authors have used 20 U botulinum toxin A injected into the glabella and forehead. This

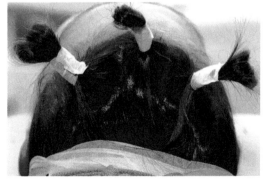

Fig. 7. Standard endoscopic brow lift surgical markings; laterally, 2 cm posterior to the temporal hairline recession, at a location demarcated by the lateral canthus and temporal line. Additionally, 2 paramedian incisions are made to gain access medially.

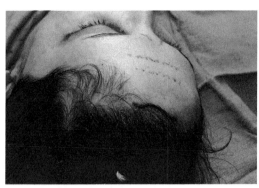

Fig. 8. The trichophytic incision is approximately 4 cm in length and is made at the midline following the natural irregular contour of the hairline. Laterally on each side a 3-cm to 4-cm incision is made 2 cm posterior to the temporal hairline recession at a location demarcated by the lateral canthus and temporal line.

combination of botulinum toxin A (Allergan, Irvine, CA) chemical ablation of the depressor muscles with planned myotomies of the depressor muscles during the endoscopic forehead lift was thought to act synergistically to maintain the elevated forehead position, and also treat the nasoglabellar furrows.[7] Recently, in an unpublished retrospective review of 464 patients, Waters and Perkins (H.H.W. and S.W.P., unpublished data, 2014) concluded the intraoperative or postoperative addition of botulinum toxin does not appear to play a significant role in the maintenance of brow elevation after endoscopic brow lifts. The incision sites and areas of planned undermining are then infiltrated with 1% lidocaine with epinephrine (1:50,000) and the forehead infiltrated with 0.5% lidocaine with epinephrine (1:100,000).

If the technique includes a trichophytic incision, for those patients with high hairlines, an incision that is approximately 4 cm in length is made at the midline following the natural irregular frontal hairline contour in a scalloped fashion, with an appropriate bevel to avoid injury to the hair follicles (see **Fig. 9**).

Laterally, in all cases, on each side, a 3-cm to 4-cm vertical incision is made 2 cm posterior to the temporal hairline recession at a location demarcated by the lateral canthus and temporal line (see **Fig. 8**). Initially, flap elevation is made in a subgaleal plane (**Fig. 10**). The posterior elevation is performed approximately 10 cm posterior to the incision sites. The posterior elevation not only minimizes the development of scalp rolls, but also mobilizes the posterior flap, allowing for closure of the trichophytic incisions while minimizing any elevation of the hairline. The temporal region is elevated in a plane between the temporoparietal fascia and the superficial layer of the deep

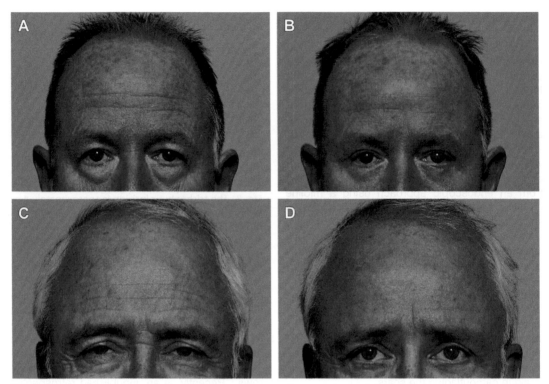

Fig. 9. (*A*) Preoperative photo of male patient with prominent androgenic alopecia, brow ptosis, and distinct forehead rhytids. (*B*) Patient 18 months postoperative from upper and lower lid blepharoplasty and combination midline transverse forehead incision and endoscopic approach brow lift with inconspicuous scar. (*C*) Male patient with significant recession of the anterior hairline, brow ptosis, and dermatochalasis. (*D*) Patient 12 months postoperative from upper and lower lid blepharoplasty and combination midline transverse forehead incision and endoscopic approach brow lift with inconspicuous scar.

temporal fascia, and the conjoint tendon is then divided (**Fig. 11**). Dissection of this temporal region is performed down to an area slightly superior to the zygomatic arch and lateral canthus. By maintaining the plane of dissection between the temporoparietal fascia and the superficial layer of the deep temporal fascia, the frontal branch of the facial nerve is protected and should be superficial to the dissection.

Following this, elevation is made in a subperiosteal plane down to a level of 2 cm above the supraorbital rim (**Fig. 12**). Arcus marginalis elevation is

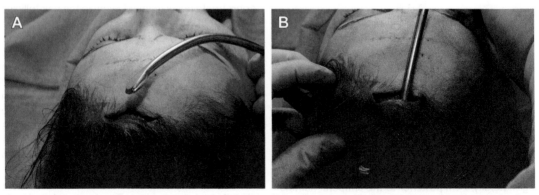

Fig. 10. (A)The Ramirez Endo Forehead parietal elevator (SnowdenPencer, Tucker, GA) is used to elevate the forehead and temporal skin in a subgaleal plane. (*B*) The elevation is continued approximately 10 cm posterior to the incision sites.

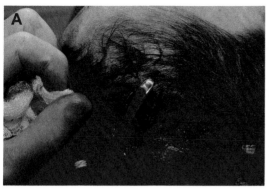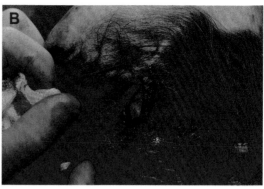

Fig. 11. (*A*) A custom-made curved elevator is positioned into the temporal region through the lateral incision to divide the conjoint tendon. (*B*) Dissection of this temporal region is performed down to an area slightly superior to the zygomatic arch and lateral canthus.

performed with the nondominant hand functioning as a guide to the level of the supraorbital rim and the location of the supraorbital foramina is palpated (**Fig. 13**). Laterally, the subperiosteal dissection is carried along the lateral orbital rim, taking care to avoid the lateral canthal tendon insertions. This elevation is performed in the region of the glabella down to the nasion. Once the arcus marginalis is elevated, an endoscope is used to provide visualization; and using a suction elevator, the inferior conjoint tendon is delineated and further divided with curved endoscopic scissors (Accurate Surgical and Scientific Instruments Corp, Westbury, NY) down to the level of the sentinel vein (**Fig. 14**). Endoscopically, the subperiosteal elevation is completed at the level of the supraorbital rim using the Isse elevator (Karl Storz, Culver City, CA) (**Fig. 15**). Care is then taken to identify and preserve the supraorbital neurovascular bundle. With a custom-made reusable electrode knife tip, the periosteum is incised in a horizontal direction at the level of the supraorbital rim (**Fig. 16**).

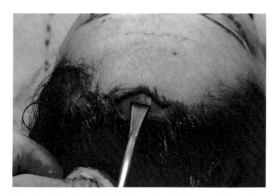

Fig. 12. The Daniel Endo Forehead elevator (Snowden Pencer) is used to elevate in a subperiosteal plane down to a level 2 cm above the supraorbital rim.

Myotomies of the corrugator supercilii and procerus muscles are performed with the electrode knife tip. Because the motor nerve to the corrugator supercilii muscle runs within the substance of the lateral orbicularis oculi muscle, we perform a lateral myotomy of the orbicularis oculi muscle not only to weaken the orbicularis oculi muscle but also to interrupt the innervation to the corrugator supercilii muscle.

If a trichophytic incision is used, an effort to camouflage the incision is made by beveling the incision, as well as deepithelializing the posterior flap. A 2-mm to 3-mm strip of epidermis from the posterior flap is excised (**Fig. 17**). The anterior flap of the trichophytic incision is lifted up, and vertical incisions are made through the anterior flap. Staples are placed at these positions to approximate the anterior and posterior flaps. The excess skin and soft tissue from the anterior flap are then excised in a beveled manner; the bevel is directed from posterior to anterior (**Fig. 18**). The staples are then removed and hemostasis is achieved with bipolar electrocautery.

Suture fixation of the flaps is accomplished via bone tunnels at the level of the outer cortex of the skull. The bone tunnels are made with the Browlift Bone Bridge system (Medtronic Xomed Surgical Products, Jacksonville, FL) and a drill bit with a 2-mm diameter and 25-mm guard (**Fig. 19**). Two bone tunnels are created at the trichophytic incision site in a horizontal direction, whereas bone tunnels are created in the vertical direction at the lateral incisions or for the standard endoscopic paramedian incisions (see **Fig. 19**). Using the drill bit with a 25-mm guard, there have been no instances of cerebrospinal fluid leaks or other intracranial complications. If significant bleeding is encountered from the bone tunnel site, hemostasis is achieved with Bone Wax

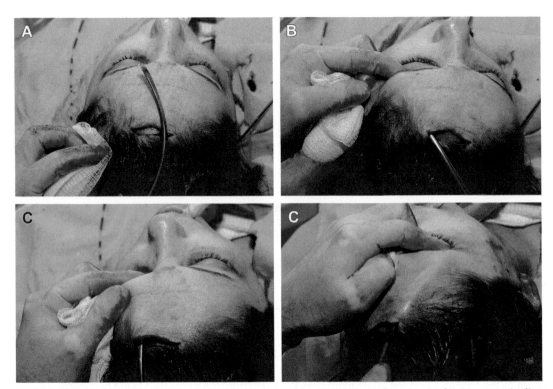

Fig. 13. (*A*) The Ramirez Endo Forehead A/M dissector (Snowden Pencer) is used to elevate the arcus marginalis at the level of the supraorbital rim. (*B–D*) The elevation is performed with the nondominant hand functioning as a guide to the level of the supraorbital rim, lateral rim, and the location of the supraorbital foramina.

(Ethicon, Somerville, NJ), and new bone tunnels are created.

A 2–0 polyglactin suture (Vicryl; Ethicon, Somerville, NJ) is used for fixation from the bone tunnel to the galea and subcutaneous tissue of the anterior

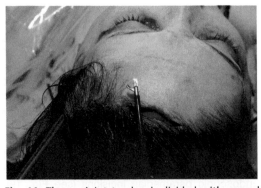

Fig. 14. The conjoint tendon is divided with curved endoscopic scissors (Accurate Surgical and Scientific Instruments Corp). This aspect of the procedure is performed under endoscopic visualization using a 30-degree endoscope, which is placed through the lateral incision.

flap to stabilize and achieve lifting of the medial forehead at the trichophytic or paramedian incision sites. Very minimal lifting is performed medially so that the medial brow may remain at the level of the supraorbital rim. The lateral forehead is lifted with the suture from the bone tunnel to the galea and the subcutaneous tissue at the most anterior aspect of the lateral incision on both sides (**Fig. 20**). This suture not only lifts the lateral forehead but also acts to reapproximate the edges of the incision. The lateral and paramedian incisions are closed with staples.

If a trichophytic incision is needed, then the closure begins in a layered fashion with 3–0 long-lasting braided absorbable suture in the deep layers, 4–0 long-lasting absorbable monofilament suture in the deep and fine dermis, and 6–0 nonabsorbable monofilament suture to further evert the cuticular edges (**Fig. 21**). With meticulous closure, the trichophytic incision is well camouflaged (**Fig. 22**).

Combination Technique

Patients with hairlines that prevent a standard endoscopic approach may benefit from a

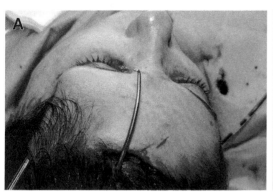
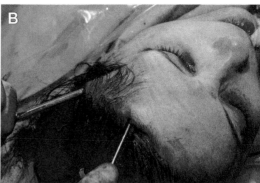

Fig. 15. (A) The subperiosteal elevation is completed at the level of the supraorbital rim using the Isse elevator. (B) The trichophytic incision provides easy access to the level of the supraorbital rim despite the high anterior hairline and double convexity of the forehead.

combination procedure using a midline transverse mid-forehead incision to address medial brow ptosis. The lateral endoscopic techniques are performed in an identical fashion as described previously.

The modified mid-forehead lift begins with a #15 blade to make an incision in a prominent transverse forehead rhytid. Dissection should be carried down in a subperiosteal plane directly in the midline, as would normally be performed in our trichophytic approach. Maintenance of this plane and staying in the midline avoids any injury to the neurovascular bundles. Hemostasis is obtained using a bipolar cautery. The inferior dissection is then carried down to the level of the superior orbital rim and nasion, exposing the corrugator and procerus muscles. Myotomies of the corrugator supercilii and procerus muscles are performed with the electrode knife tip or performed sharply. The superior skin flap is back elevated for a distance of 1 cm.

The subcutaneous and subdermal layers are re-approximated using interrupted 5–0 resorbable monofilament suture. The fine dermis is closed with a 6–0 absorbable Polysorb suture (Covidien, Mansfield, MA) and the cuticular edges everted using a running 6–0 polypropylene subcuticular suture. The ends of the sutures were then secured using adhesive strips. Because of the risk of visible scars, eversion is necessary, and several interrupted 6–0 mild chromic sutures can be placed to further evert the skin edges. With meticulous closure, the transverse forehead incisions can heal in an inconspicuous fashion (**Fig. 23**).

POSTPROCEDURAL CARE

After upper facial rejuvenation, patients are counseled to continue with a strict eye moisturization protocol when blepharoplasty is part of their surgical treatment. This involves ocular lubrication with artificial tears every hour, gel lubricant while

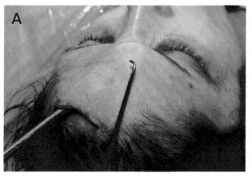
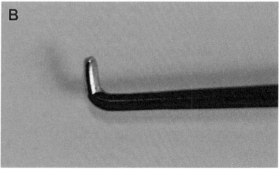

Fig. 16. (A) Custom-made reusable electrode knife tip is used to incise the periosteum and perform myotomies of the corrugator supercilii and procerus muscles. (B) Custom-made guarded reusable electrode knife tip.

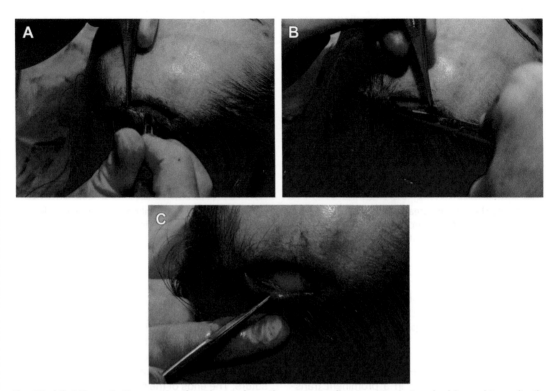

Fig. 17. (*A*) A 2-mm to 3-mm strip of epidermis from the posterior flap is excised. A scalpel is used to make the incision through the epidermis. (*B*) Sharp curved scissors are then used to complete the excision of the strip of epidermis. (*C*) The intact dermis, subcutaneous tissue, and hair follicles after removal of the epidermal layer.

sleeping, and antibiotic ointment along the incision lines 4 times daily after cleansing with hydrogen peroxide on a cotton tip applicator.

After an endoscopic brow lift, a light compressive head wrap dressing is left in place for 24 hours, and all patients are seen on postoperative day 1 where the wrap is removed. We instruct all patients to wash their hair daily with gentle shampoo until all sutures and staples are removed on postoperative day 7. A complimentary esthetic session is provided to patients who have had eyelid surgery to cover any ecchymosis that may be visible. Activity restrictions remain in place for 2 weeks and patients are reminded to not rub the eyes for several weeks until all upper eyelid incisions have completely healed. Additionally, because of the expected hypesthesia after brow lift procedures, patients are instructed to avoid, or carefully use, curling irons, hair dryers, or any potential thermal or chemical irritation to the scalp or forehead.

COMPLICATIONS (AND THEIR MANAGEMENT)

Avoiding and managing complications in the setting of surgical periorbital rejuvenation is discussed in detail earlier in this issue. We highlight the complications specific to upper lid blepharoplasty and brow lift procedures.

Upper Lid Blepharoplasty

During upper eyelid blepharoplasty, duteous hemostasis is of utmost importance not only to maintain a clear operative field but also to minimize the risk of postoperative bleeding. Hematomas are rare, but if present, they are often simply a subcutaneous collection, making drainage, if necessary, as simple as opening the incision, obtaining hemostasis, and suturing the incision closed. With any eyelid surgery, there is the potential risk of lagophthalmos; however, with maintaining a conservative approach when marking the patient, as described previously, the risk of skin over-resection is insignificant, and the likelihood of conspicuous scarring is minimized as well by following these guidelines. Fat resection during upper lid blepharoplasty can lead to hollowing, effectively aging the patient further within the upper third of the face. The surgeon should be cognizant of this potential, and if encountered, adjunctive procedures with fillers or

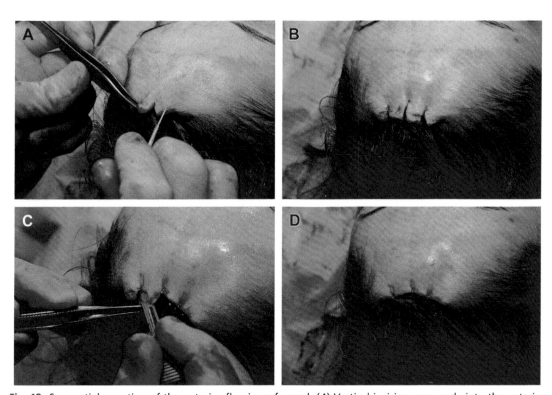

Fig. 18. Sequential resection of the anterior flap is performed. (*A*) Vertical incisions are made into the anterior flap, and (*B*) staples are placed to approximate the anterior and posterior flaps. (*C*) The excess skin and soft tissue from the anterior flap is then excised in a beveled (posterior to anterior) manner. (*D*) The result after this skin excision.

autologous fat grafting should be considered to correct the deformity.

Forehead and Brow Lifting

After forehead or brow lifting, the undermined areas produce a space for fluid to accumulate. The light compressive head wrap described previously is fashioned from a gauze roll, and helps to minimize any blood or serous fluid collection within this space. This is quite effective in reducing the incidence of hematomas, and there is very little discomfort to the patient, given the short period of wearing the wrap. Hematomas are rare, but

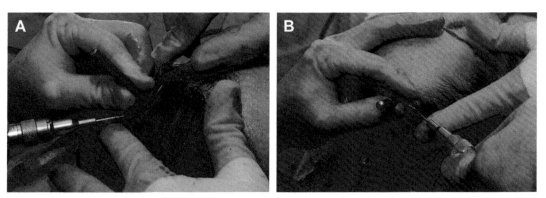

Fig. 19. (*A*) The Browlift Bone Bridge system (Medtronic Xomed Surgical Products) and drill bit with a 2-mm diameter and a 25-mm guard is used to make a vertically oriented tunnel at the lateral incision. (*B*) Two horizontally oriented bone tunnels are made at the trichophytic incision.

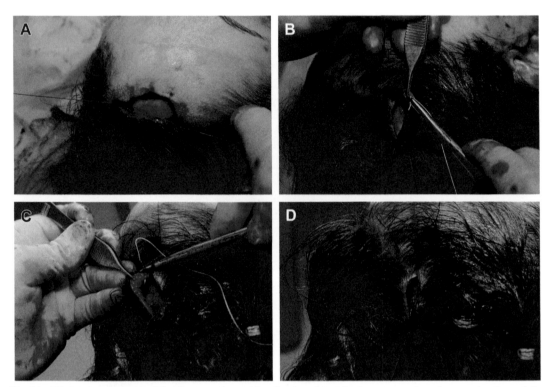

Fig. 20. (*A*) A 2–0 polyglactin (Vicryl) suture is used for fixation from the bone tunnel to the anterior flap of the trichophytic incision. (*B, C*) At the lateral incision, fixation is achieved with suture from the bone tunnel to the most anterior aspect of the lateral incision on both sides. (*D*) This suture not only lifts the lateral forehead but also acts to reapproximate the edges of the lateral incision. The suture is passed through galea to achieve proper tissue strength for elevation and fixation.

if encountered, needle aspiration should be attempted in the office setting. If a hematoma is persistent or congealed, opening the incision, draining the collection, and reapplying the head wrap may be necessary. The authors have not had to return to the operating room for evacuation of hematoma after an endoscopic brow procedure.

Hypesthesia is a known temporary sequela following brow rejuvenation, and in some instances alopecia can be seen. The surgeon should reassure the patient that both of these concerns, if present, are only transient, and full recovery should be expected in the next several months. Also, given the scalp numbness, the surgeon should reiterate the necessary lifestyle modifications and thermal precautions, discussed previously, until sensation returns.

Injury to the facial nerve during an endoscopic brow lift is a dreaded complication, but fortunately of rare incidence. A thorough understanding of the anatomy, and relationship of the facial nerve to the sentinel vein, is critical to maintain the correct plane of dissection and avoid damaging the nerve. Thought to be more common than direction

transection, stretch injury to the nerve can occur if too much pressure is applied on the flap with the endoscope, and the surgeon should be sensitive to the amount of force used for visualization.

The disadvantages and complications of the trichophytic or transverse mid-forehead incisions include the potential for depigmented or widened scars with resulting visible cosmetic deformity, as well an increased operative time, and potential larger area of hypesthesia with the trichophytic incision. Prominent scarring can be minimized with use of a meticulous technique and closure as described previously. Other concerns include brow asymmetry, which may be preexisting, due to poor marking, or as a result of suture failure during the suspension, and can be quite difficult to correct.

OUTCOMES

Attention to the upper third of the face and periorbital region is essential to any well-balanced facial rejuvenation. With advances in technology and techniques, the endoscopic approach to forehead

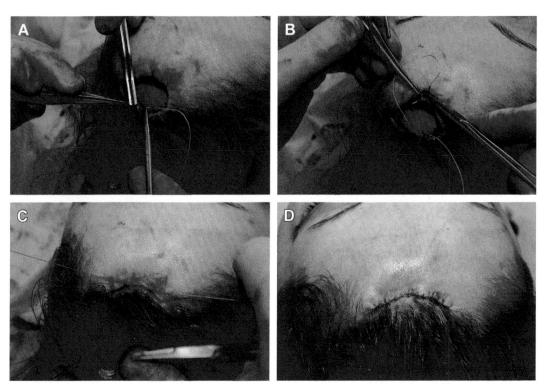

Fig. 21. (*A, B*) Meticulous closure of the trichophytic incision is performed with a 3–0 polyglactin suture in an interrupted buried fashion to obtain deep-tissue approximation. (*C*) The assistant further mobilizes the posterior flap to allow closure of the wound without moving the hairline more posteriorly. Further subcutaneous approximation is achieved with 4–0 polydioxanone. (*D*) After this maneuver, skin closure with proper eversion of the skin edges is achieved with a 6–0 blue polypropylene suture in a running interlocked manner.

and brow lifting has gained acceptance as the ideal surgical management of the upper third of the face, with concomitant upper lid blepharoplasty when indicated. Initially, this approach was met with resistance because of the learning curve and specialized equipment necessary to achieve consistent outcomes, with several discussions regarding the ideal dissection plane, longevity, and method of fixation.[15–17]

The debates have spurred surgeons to form unique research tools to accurately quantify

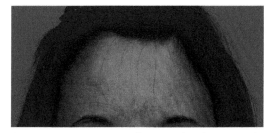

Fig. 22. Postoperative photograph showing the esthetic result of the trichophytic incision at 12 months.

esthetic changes in the upper face when comparing techniques, methods of fixation, and results, including longevity.[18] Several investigators have used fixed anatomic points as references to quantify outcomes, including calibrating the diameter of the iris, or drawing perpendicular lines at the level of the lateral canthus, medial canthus, midpupillary line, and the midpoints between the pupil and the lateral and medial canthi to standardize measurements.[19,20] Papadopulos and colleagues[21] retrospectively reviewed 98 patients using similar measurement criteria showing long-lasting results with high patient satisfaction. Kim and colleagues[22] compared the preoperative and postoperative ratio of the vertical distance between the lateral corneal limbus and the superior brow and the horizontal distance between the lateral limbus and the medial canthus, reporting long-term brow elevation using endoscopic techniques. Waters and Perkins (H.H.W. and S.W.P., unpublished data, 2014) performed a large retrospective study evaluating 464 consecutive patients, further validating the long-term results in correction of the aging upper third of the face using the endoscopic techniques described herein,

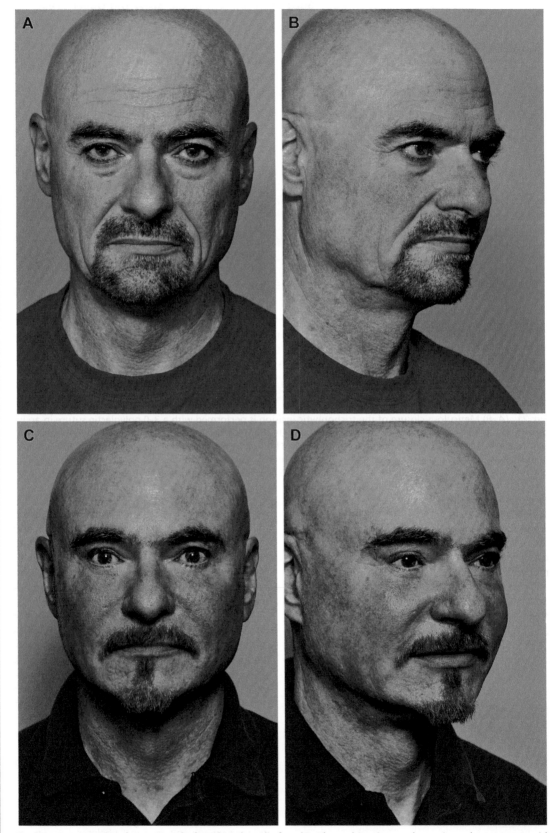

Fig. 23. An example of a patient before (*A*, *B*) and after (*C*, *D*) combination endoscopic and transverse mid-forehead lift. The patient underwent concomitant upper and lower lid blepharoplasty and later rhytidectomy and is 30 months postoperative from upper facial rejuvenation.

with dissection in the subperiosteal plane and bone bridge fixation.

SUMMARY

Surgical management of the aging upper face continues to take on a central role in total facial rejuvenation, with a variety of techniques available. The endoscopic brow lift uses short incisions; is safe, long-lasting, and easily implemented; and with the combination techniques has new-found expansion in its indications. The upper facial structures should be assessed individually and as part of the brow-eyelid continuum to guide selection of the appropriate treatments that will meet the esthetic goals of the patient and surgeon alike.

ACKNOWLEDGMENTS

The authors acknowledge Nancy A. Rothrock for her assistance in the preparation of the digital images used in this article.

REFERENCES

1. Czyz CN, Hill RH, Foster JA. Preoperative evaluation of the brow-lid continuum. Clin Plast Surg 2013; 40(1):43–53.
2. Donath AS, Glasgold RA, Glasgold MJ. Volume loss versus gravity: new concepts in facial aging. Curr Opin Otolaryngol Head Neck Surg 2007;15(4):238–43.
3. Lam VB, Czyz CN, Wulc AE. The brow-eyelid continuum: an anatomic perspective. Clin Plast Surg 2013; 40(1):1–19.
4. Fitzgerald R. Contemporary concepts in brow and eyelid aging. Clin Plast Surg 2013;40(1):21–42.
5. Lambros V. Observations on periorbital and midface aging. Plast Reconstr Surg 2007;120(5):1367–76 [discussion: 1377].
6. Friedman O. Changes associated with the aging face. Facial Plast Surg Clin North Am 2005;13(3): 371–80.
7. Batniji RK, Perkins SW. Upper and midfacial rejuvenation in the non-Caucasian face. Facial Plast Surg Clin North Am 2010;18(1):19–33.
8. Gunter JP, Antrobus SD. Aesthetic analysis of the eyebrows. Plast Reconstr Surg 1997;99(7):1808–16.
9. Chand M, Perkins SW. Comparison of surgical approaches for upper facial rejuvenation. Curr Opin Otolaryngol Head Neck Surg 2000;8(4):326–31.
10. Kerth JD, Toriumi DM. Management of the aging forehead. Arch Otolaryngol Head Neck Surg 1990; 116(10):1137–42.
11. Pitanguy I. Section of the frontalis-procerus-corrugator aponeurosis in the correction of frontal and glabellar wrinkles. Ann Plast Surg 1979;2(5): 422–7.
12. Javidnia H, Sykes J. Endoscopic brow lifts: have they replaced coronal lifts? Facial Plast Surg Clin North Am 2013;21(2):191–9.
13. Lambros V. Volumizing the brow with hyaluronic acid fillers. Aesthet Surg J 2009;29(3):174–9.
14. Buckingham ED, Bader B, Smith SP. Autologous fat and fillers in periocular rejuvenation. Facial Plast Surg Clin North Am 2010;18(3):385–98.
15. Dayan SH, Perkins SW, Vartanian AJ, et al. The forehead lift: endoscopic versus coronal approaches. Aesthetic Plast Surg 2001;25(1):35–9.
16. Chiu ES, Baker DC. Endoscopic brow lift: a retrospective review of 628 consecutive cases over 5 years. Plast Reconstr Surg 2003;112(2):628–33 [discussion: 634–5].
17. Elkwood A, Matarasso A, Rankin M, et al. National plastic surgery survey: brow lifting techniques and complications. Plast Reconstr Surg 2001;108(7): 2143–50 [discussion: 2151–2].
18. Romo T 3rd, Zoumalan RA, Rafii BY. Current concepts in the management of the aging forehead in facial plastic surgery. Curr Opin Otolaryngol Head Neck Surg 2010;18(4):272–7.
19. Graf RM, Tolazzi AR, Mansur AE, et al. Endoscopic periosteal brow lift: evaluation and follow-up of eyebrow height. Plast Reconstr Surg 2008;121(2): 609–16 [discussion: 617–9].
20. Badin AZ, Bittencourt LM, Balderrama CR. Lateral brow fixation in endoscopic forehead lift: long-term results with braided nylon percutaneous sutures. Aesthetic Plast Surg 2010;34(1):78–87.
21. Papadopulos NA, Eder M, Weigand C, et al. A review of 13 years of experience with endoscopic forehead-lift. Arch Facial Plast Surg 2012;14(5): 336–41.
22. Kim BP, Goode RL, Newman JP. Brow elevation ratio: a new method of brow analysis. Arch Facial Plast Surg 2009;11(1):34–9.

Midface Skeletal Enhancement

Danny J. Soares, MD[a], William E. Silver, MD[b,c],*

KEYWORDS

- Alloplastic malar augmentation • Midface surgery • Midface augmentation • Cheek augmentation
- Cheek implants

KEY POINTS

- Alloplastic malar augmentation provides a permanent yet reversible form of midfacial rejuvenation that can be tailored to patients' anatomy.
- Malar deformities can be categorized into types I, II, and III, depending on the presence of bony malar hypoplasia, submalar soft tissue volume loss/ptosis, or both, respectively.
- Choosing the correct implant design is essential in achieving ideal malar augmentation. A combination of malar, submalar, and malar-submalar implant shapes are available.
- The surgeon should thoroughly inspect the face for the presence of any significant preexisting facial asymmetries before determining the type and size of implant to be used.
- The transoral surgical approach allows for rapid and precise placement of malar implants. Implant stabilization in the immediate postoperative period is necessary to minimize the possibility of implant displacement.

A video of midface skeletal enhancement accompanies this article at http://www.facialplastic. theclinics.com/

INTRODUCTION

The malar region may be considered the most important facial region imparting a youthful countenance to the human visage. The combination of the underlying bony support, adipose tissue, and mimetic musculature generates a dynamic dimension to the face that is essential for the beauty of human expression and facial balance. Such a delicate arrangement is prone to deformation because of the ever-present forces of aging, gravity, solar radiation, and bodyweight fluctuations. Over time, even a full malar pad becomes ptotic and atrophic, leading to the withered appearance characteristic of senescence. The presence of additional congenital malar bony deficiency accentuates such aging changes and may even act to accelerate them.

Presently, the modern facial aesthetic surgeon has an available surgical and nonsurgical arsenal that is unmatched compared with any other period in the history of our field. According to the American Society of Plastic Surgeons, as of 2013, hyaluronic acid augmentation of the face has risen to become the second most commonly performed nonsurgical procedure in the United States, behind only botulinum toxin, with nearly 2 million procedures performed yearly.[1] Such rapid growth

Disclosures: The authors have no disclosures to make.
[a] Private Practice, Mesos Plastic & Laser Surgery, 757 County Road 466, Lady Lake, FL 32159, USA; [b] Department of Otolaryngology, Head & Neck Surgery, Emory University, Atlanta, GA 30322, USA; [c] Private Practice, Premier Image Cosmetic & Laser Surgery, 4553 North Shallowford Road, Suite 20-B, Atlanta, GA 30338, USA
* Corresponding author. Emory University, Department of Otolaryngology, Head & Neck Surgery, Atlanta, GA 30322.
E-mail address: wesilver@me.com

Facial Plast Surg Clin N Am 23 (2015) 185–193
http://dx.doi.org/10.1016/j.fsc.2015.01.004
1064-7406/15/$ – see front matter © 2015 Elsevier Inc. All rights reserved.

and widespread use have been fueled by a need to create a more balanced, fuller, and, therefore, youthful facial harmony via augmentation of the cheeks. Despite this, injectable midface augmentation has shown limitations with durability, permissibility of large-volume augmentation, and correction of bony malar deficiency without imparting an adynamic or bloated-face appearance. Alloplastic augmentation provides a durable yet reversible form of malar augmentation that lends itself well to a significant proportion of patients seeking midfacial volume enhancement. This article describes the intrinsic details inherent to alloplastic midfacial augmentation, with procedural details describing the most commonly used surgical technique in current use.

TREATMENT GOALS AND PLANNED OUTCOMES

The primary goal of alloplastic midface augmentation is to attain a permanent volumetric enhancement of one or more components of the malar region, with a secondary endeavor to achieve an improved degree of facial symmetry. Anatomically, the *malar eminence* is the most protuberant bony prominence of the midface and represents the body of the zygomatic bone, which can be easily palpated on physical examination. The presence of bony hypoplasia imparts a certain degree of *flatness* to the human face that can be easily identified and should be carefully noted preoperatively. Measuring the bizygomatic distance on a frontal view can aid in the identification of malar hypoplasia, as that value typically exceeds the bigonial distance by 25% to 30% in patients with aesthetically balanced faces (**Fig. 1**).[2]

A second distinct region of the midface, the *submalar triangle*, is defined as the region bordered superiorly by the malar eminence, medially by the nasofacial fold, and laterally by the masseter muscle. This region is essential to consider before cheek augmentation, as this region's apparent fullness primarily depends on its soft tissue content, in particular the malar fat pad. During the process of natural aging or in those affected by lipodystrophy of the midface, the submalar triangle undergoes significant volume loss secondary to adipose tissue atrophy and/or midfacial soft tissue ptosis. The presence of significant submalar volume loss indicates the need for a cheek implant design that specifically augments this region.[3]

Patients seeking malar augmentation have previously undergone multiple rounds of cheek volume enhancement via injection with one of the currently available temporary fillers. Often, these individuals prefer the convenience and cost-

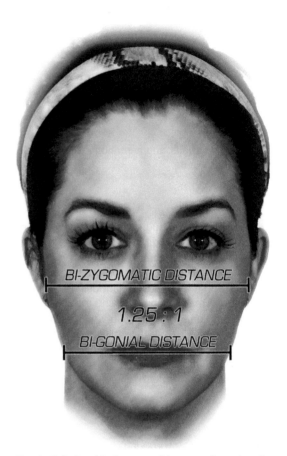

Fig. 1. Relationship between bizygomatic and malar distances. A ratio of 1.25:1.0 traditionally exists between these two distances but is often closer to 1:1 in individuals with malar hypoplasia or prominent gonial angles.

effectiveness of a one-time procedure for long-lasting augmentation. Surgically, the placement of a solid implant directly on a hypoplastic bony malar region also yields a more natural result that easily achieves a high degree of aesthetic enhancement. Despite these truths, the aesthetic facial surgeon should consider a multitude of patient and implant features before recommending this procedure to cosmetic patients.

PREOPERATIVE PLANNING AND PREPARATION
Implant Design

The extent of the midfacial augmentation as it relates to implant shape and size largely depends on the physical examination findings and the apparent degree of bony and soft tissue deficiencies of the malar region. As originally described by Binder,[4] 3 types of midface deformity can exist, which are classified into types I, II, and III (**Fig. 2**). Individuals with a type I deformity

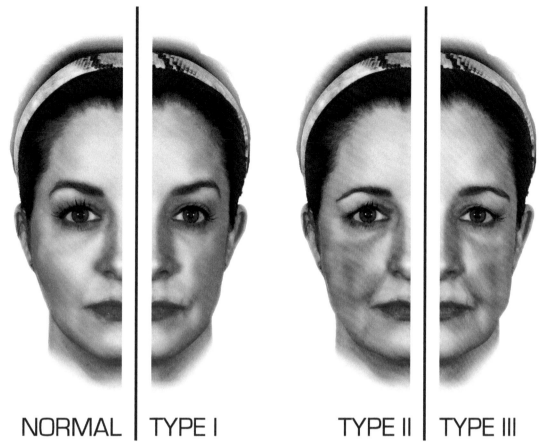

NORMAL | TYPE I   TYPE II | TYPE III

Fig. 2. Binder classification of midface deformities. Type I patients demonstrate mostly malar bony hypoplasia with otherwise normal submalar soft tissue pad. Individuals with type II cheeks have normal bony eminences but loss of submalar soft tissue volume caused by aging-related volume loss and ptosis or primary adipose tissue loss from lipodystrophy. Type III patients have a combination of bony hypoplasia and submalar soft tissue volume loss. (*From* Silver W, Soares D. Facial contouring with implants. In: Sclafani A, editor. Facial plastic and reconstructive surgery. In: Sataloff R, editor. Sataloff's comprehensive textbook of otolaryngology. Philadelphia: JP Brothers Medical Publishers; 2014. p. 15; with permission.)

display a certain degree of malar bony hypoplasia but otherwise have relatively normal midfacial soft tissue volumes. Type I patients benefit from the insertion of a *malar*-type implant (**Fig. 3**). Patients with a type II deformity, the most commonly encountered form, have normally projecting malar bony eminences but demonstrate considerable midfacial soft tissue loss caused by fat atrophy and/or malar ptosis, often secondary to the aging process. These patients require the insertion of a *submalar*-type implant, which specifically augments the submalar triangle (see **Fig. 3**). Finally, those with a type III midface deformity have a combination of both malar bony hypoplasia and soft tissue loss or ptosis. Type III individuals benefit most from a combined *malar-submalar*–type implant (see **Fig. 3**). Once the ideal implant design is chosen, the surgeon should next determine which implant material to use.

Implant Material

Although the ideal implant material is yet to be discovered, the few that do exist currently have well-established track records of safety and durability in addition to the necessary mechanical qualities for aesthetic facial augmentation. A variety of different implant materials are available for malar augmentation, each with their own specific benefits and disadvantages.[5,6]

Silicone implants (Implantech, Ventura, CA) are composed of vulcanized dimethylsiloxane polymer, which yields a pliable rubber that is nonporous and easily adapted for facial contouring. Silicone rubber implants are remarkably resistant to enzymatic breakdown and autoclaving, lack significant tissue immunogenicity, and are well tolerated by robustly vascularized recipient tissues. Because of their nonporous nature, silicone

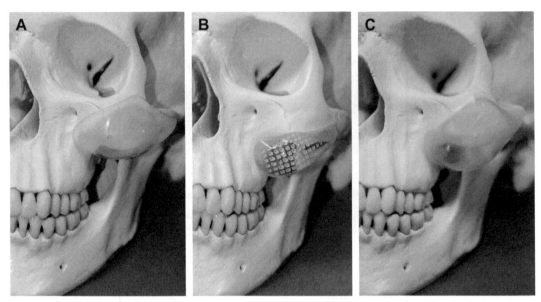

Fig. 3. Types of preformed malar implants. (*A*) Malar. (*B*) Submalar. (*C*) Combined malar-submalar. (*From* Silver W, Soares D. Facial contouring with implants. In: Sclafani A, editor. Facial plastic and reconstructive surgery. In: Sataloff R, editor. Sataloff's comprehensive textbook of otolaryngology. Philadelphia: JP Brothers Medical Publishers; 2014. p. 15; with permission.)

rubber implants do not allow for tissue ingrowth and, thus, incite a significant degree of capsular formation that actually aids in implant stabilization. However, the lack of any tissue ingrowth can mean that the implant may be easily displaced in the immediate postoperative period, if it is not sufficiently stabilized, before capsule formation has occurred, and may also be prone to deformation over time due to tissue contraction. Fortunately, when applied against the firm midfacial bony structure of the maxillary and zygomatic bones, it provides a relatively stable augmentation without significant implant deformation or displacement after healing has occurred.

The microporous expanded polytetrafluoroethylene implant material (ePTFE; *Gore-tex*, W.L. Gore and Associates, Flagstaff, AZ) is a versatile option available for malar augmentation. With pore sizes in the range of 10 to 30 μm, ePTFE implants allow for a small amount of tissue ingrowth that helps to stabilize the implant without creating the often difficult task of implant removal, should the need arise, that is often seen with macroporous implant materials. ePTFE is also easily accepted by well-vascularized facial tissues and also does not display any degree of tissue toxicity or immunogenicity.

Macroporous alloplastic implants, such as high-density polyethylene (Medpor, Porex Surgical Inc, College Park, GA), are characterized by pore sizes of 125 to 250 μm and, thus, allow for a large degree of tissue ingrowth. This feature results in rapid implant stabilization and may even reduce the incidence of implant infection secondary to improved vascularization of the implant–soft tissue interface. However, once tissue ingrowth has occurred, implant removal may be laborious and could require the excision of a cuff of normal recipient tissue along with the implant.

Preoperative Patient Preparation

Patients wishing to undergo alloplastic malar augmentation should be well informed of the intrinsic risks and benefits of the procedure, including the risk of complications relating to implant insertion, such as infection, extrusion, displacement, deformation, and motor and sensory nerve injury, as well as the risks of the desired level of anesthesia. In addition, patients should be screened for any active or prior history of immunosuppression, connective tissue disorders, coagulopathy, facial trauma, and implanted facial hardware, among others, before being deemed fit for the procedure. In addition, patients should also be inquired regarding any recent injections of permanent or temporary fillers (especially high volume), as these may interfere with the ability to proceed with surgery or achieve an ideal result. Standard preoperative photography should be obtained as with any other facial cosmetic procedure. Finally, preexisting facial asymmetries should be noted before surgery and discussed thoroughly with patients. Often, preexisting facial asymmetries will be augmented if the surgeon does not recognize and address this problem intraoperatively. Placing implants of different sizes, or performing custom implant carving, will help correct any significant malar imbalance.

PATIENT POSITIONING

Patients are placed in a sitting position for the preoperative marking to ensure that an unnatural gravity vector does not distort all landmarks and delineated areas to be augmented. Patients are placed in a supine position for the actual surgical procedure.

PROCEDURAL APPROACH
Preoperative Marking

Before surgical malar augmentation, the malar region should be outlined with patients in a sitting position to facilitate symmetric placement of the malar implants (Video 1). Tracing the location of the inferior orbital rim and the infraorbital foramina will also aid in avoiding injury to nearby structures. Constructing Silver's malar prominence triangle (Fig. 4) will assist with all of those tasks. The size and shape of the implant should also be delineated on the skin to help prevent the creation of an excessively large pocket, which can predispose to implant displacement postoperatively. The infraorbital neurovascular bundle and foramina should be located and marked, serving as the medial-most extent of the dissection. Superiorly, tissue dissection should not proceed beyond the inferior orbital rim, as this could lead to a lower-lid contour deformity secondary to superior displacement of the implant.

Surgical technique
This surgical procedure can be easily performed under either local anesthetic with or without sedation or general inhaled anesthesia. Appropriate regional nerve blockade is achieved via infiltration of 1% lidocaine with 1:100,000 epinephrine targeting the infraorbital and superior alveolar nerves. Appropriate antibiotic prophylaxis is provided 30 minutes before the incision with either intravenous cefazolin or clindamycin. Patients are then draped in the usual sterile fashion, and the skin is prepped with povidone-iodine (Betadine) solution. Next, a small incision is made with a No. 15 blade adjacent to the canine fossa, leaving at least 1.5 cm of gingival mucosa for later incisional closure. The tissue dissection is carried all the way down to the maxillary bone with monopolar electrocautery; the periosteum is subsequently

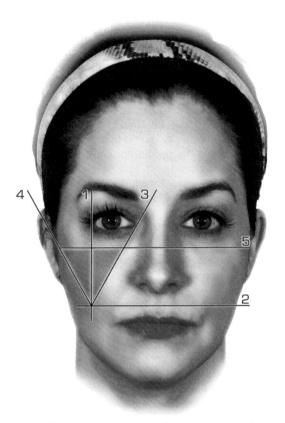

Fig. 4. Constructing Silver's malar prominence triangle. A vertical line is drawn intersecting the lateral canthus (1). A line perpendicular to (1) is drawn midway between the subnasale and upper lip vermillion border. Next, a line (3) is drawn from the medial canthus to the intersection point between (1) and (2). Line (3) is then reflected over (1), creating line (4). Lastly, the Frankfort horizontal line is drawn (5). The triangle is delineated by lines (3), (4), and (5). (From Silver W, Soares D. Facial contouring with implants. In: Sclafani A, editor. Facial plastic and reconstructive surgery. In: Sataloff R, editor. Sataloff's comprehensive textbook of otolaryngology. Philadelphia: JP Brothers Medical Publishers; 2014. p. 14; with permission.)

incised; subperiosteal dissection is then carefully undertaken with an elevator. It is important to always keep the location of the infraorbital nerve and inferior orbital rim under palpation as one creates the subperiosteal pocket. The surgeon should aim to create a pocket that is only slightly larger than the implant itself but also ensure that it is in the correct configuration.

Placement of the alloplastic malar implant should be preceded by immersion of the implant within an antibiotic solution (such as 300 mg/ 15 mL clindamycin solution) in order to counteract the bacterial contamination that is inherent to the transoral route. If a porous material is to be inserted, it is wise to pressure load the material with the antibiotic solution before insertion. The implant is then guided into position with a silk suture, twice-puncturing the implant at its superior-lateral corner that is then fed through the transoral incision, aimed at the superior-lateral apex of the implant pocket, driven by a Stamey needle (CS Surgical INC, Slidell, LA) toward its exit in the temporal scalp. A stab incision is made in the scalp region overlying the needle tip, and the silk suture ends are retrieved and tied over an antibiotic-impregnated bolster for short-term implant stabilization. The intraoral incision is then closed in a 2-layered fashion with 3–0 chromic gut sutures for the muscle and mucosal layers.

POTENTIAL COMPLICATIONS AND MANAGEMENT OF THEM
Implant Displacement

Postoperative complications following malar augmentation are rare and tend to concern, for the most part, implant malposition or postoperative asymmetry. Malposition is easily prevented when good surgical technique is used; the surgeon should avoid creating an excessively large implant pocket and stabilize the implant in position with transcutaneous sutures or other fixation methods. Fortunately, given the thickness of the malar soft tissue envelope, minor implant displacements are inconsequential from an aesthetic point of view. The development of postoperative facial asymmetry is often caused by asymmetric edema and tends to resolve as the edematous phase clears over 3 to 4 weeks. The surgeon should always carefully evaluate the face before surgery to determine if significant malar asymmetry exists. Inserting implants of different sizes, or performing custom implant carving, can help correct preexisting facial asymmetries. Should a significant difference in malar contour persist even after resolution of the edematous phase, the surgeon should strongly consider surgical revision.

Infection

Infection following malar augmentation is fortunately very rare because of the robust vascular supply of the region. However, the need for a transoral route of placement renders the risk of contamination ever-present. In the rare event of implant infection following silicone implant placement, cultures should be obtained and directed antibiotic therapy instituted immediately. If a porous implant has been inserted, then immediate removal should be sought, followed by irrigation and appropriate culture-directed antibiotic

therapy. At least 6 to 8 weeks should be allowed to pass before contemplating implant reinsertion.

Nerve Injury

Motor and sensory nerve injuries are also extremely rare but possible. Awareness of the location of the infraorbital nerve and ensuring that a subperiosteal dissection is maintained will help avoid injury to the infraorbital and facial nerves, respectively. Often, even following significant neuropraxia or neurotmesis, midfacial sensory function will return. Motor nerve injury is also likely to recover because of the presence of significant redundancy of innervation in the area; the exception, of course, would be the frontal nerve, which is at risk of injury as it courses along over the zygomatic arch. Subperiosteal dissection is essential in helping to avoid injury to this very functional and aesthetic motor nerve branch.

POSTPROCEDURAL CARE

Prophylactic antibiotic coverage is provided to patients for the subsequent 5 postoperative days. The bolster and stabilizing sutures are removed on postoperative day number 3. Because of the subperiosteal dissection, patients may expect a moderate amount of facial swelling for 2 to 3 weeks after the procedure. The addition of a short course of oral steroids is often prescribed to help reduce the severity of the postoperative edema. Standard photographs are obtained at 3, 6, and 12 months following the procedure.

REHABILITATION AND RECOVERY

Alloplastic augmentation of the midface does not result in any degree of temporary physical disability; however, patients are advised to avoid any heavy lifting or exercise for the first 1 week following surgery. A certain degree of social downtime is expected to allow for most of the edema to resolve; but this is quite patient specific and, therefore, variable. Approximately 80% of patients will have complete resolution of facial edema within 3 to 4 weeks.[7] Early steroid therapy postoperatively should be considered to aid in minimizing the degree of the edematous response. A soft diet is recommended for the first 5 to 7 days to avoid incisional abrasion, as well as excessive cheek motion caused by chewing, in order to limit any chances of implant displacement.

OUTCOMES

Figs. 5 and 6 display examples of preoperative and postoperative facial views in patients having

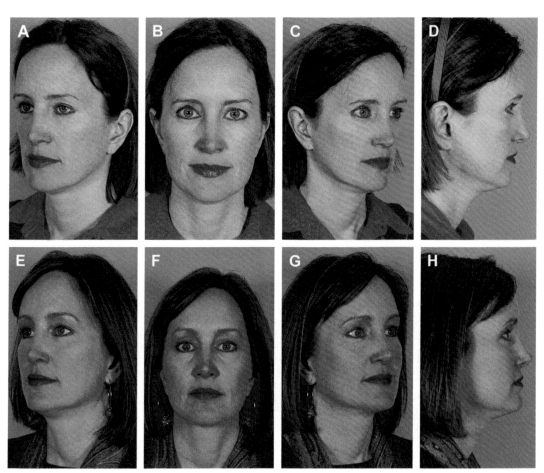

Fig. 5. Preoperative and postoperative photographs following malar augmentation. (*A–D*) Preoperative photographs displaying a patient with type I midface deformity. (*E–H*) Postoperative photographs 3 months following cheek augmentation with malar implants and endoscopic brow lift. (*From* Silver W, Soares D. Facial contouring with implants. In: Sclafani A, editor. Facial plastic and reconstructive surgery. In: Sataloff R, editor. Sataloff's comprehensive textbook of otolaryngology. Philadelphia: JP Brothers Medical Publishers; 2014. p. 17; with permission.)

undergone malar augmentation. Preoperatively, the patient shown in **Fig. 5** demonstrated a type I facial deformity and, therefore, underwent augmentation with a malar-type facial implant. The patient displayed in **Fig. 6** displayed a type II facial deformity preoperatively, characteristic of the aging face with loss and ptosis of submalar tissue. Malar augmentation in conjunction with rhytidectomy yielded a more youthful facial shape postoperatively.

CLINICAL RESULTS IN THE LITERATURE AND EVIDENCE

The wide applicability of alloplastic implants for use within the facial regions demonstrates their suitability for correction of facial volume, contour, and symmetry losses. The gradual dissipation of midfacial volume is a well-known phenomenon resulting from facial aging and is often associated with other classic aging-related changes, such as the development of the jowl, excess neck skin laxity and banding, and the deepening of the nasolabial and labiomental folds. Therefore, the modern aesthetic facial surgeon will often recommend the simultaneous coupling of midfacial alloplastic augmentation with cervicofacial rhytidectomy, periorbital rejuvenating surgery, and other procedures. Hopping and colleagues[7] reviewed 100 cases of rhytidectomy with alloplastic midface augmentation and compared it with 200 isolated rhytidectomies, finding no significant increase in procedure complications or morbidity with the addition of alloplastic malar implant placement to rhytidectomy.

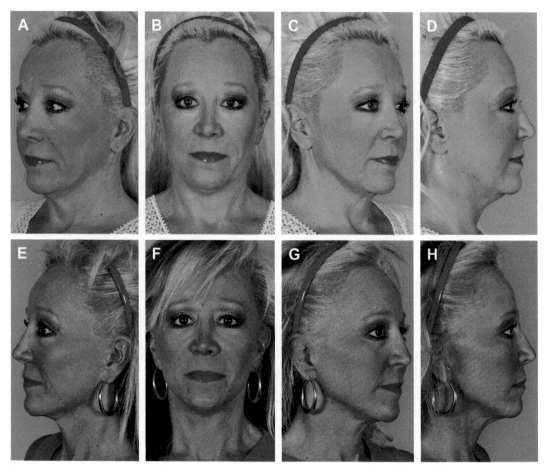

Fig. 6. Preoperative and postoperative photographs following malar augmentation and rhytidectomy. (*A–D*) Preoperative photographs displaying a patient with a type II midface deformity. (*E–H*) Postoperative photographs 17 months following cheek augmentation with submalar implants, cervicofacial rhytidectomy, and fractional carbon dioxide laser skin resurfacing. (*From* Silver W, Soares D. Facial contouring with implants. In: Sclafani A, editor. Facial plastic and reconstructive surgery. In: Sataloff R, editor. Sataloff's comprehensive textbook of otolaryngology. Philadelphia: JP Brothers Medical Publishers; 2014. p. 18; with permission.)

The use of alloplastic implants within the face has seen a variety of complications occur, such as infection, extrusion, and displacement or distortion, depending on recipient site, adequacy of soft tissue coverage, and chosen implant material. Overall, the incidences of implant infection, extrusion, and displacement within the malar region have been quoted at 2.4%, less than 0.5%, and 2.3%, respectively, with a rate of implant removal of 4.2%.[6] The thickness of midfacial tissue coverage for malar implants placed subperiosteally ensures that implant exposure and extrusion are extremely rare events. In addition, the placement of the implants against the maxillary bone helps to prevent the occurrence of implant distortion. The risk of implant displacement is minimized by the placement of fixation sutures, with different transcutaneous methods available.[4]

SUMMARY

Malar augmentation with alloplastic implants continues to serve as a reliable method of achieving a permanent yet reversible form of midfacial volume enhancement and rejuvenation. The procedure allows for placement of different implant shapes to correct different types of malar deformities. The insertion of malar implants provides the necessary volume to correct underlying congenital asymmetries, malar hypoplasia, or soft tissue volume loss and ptosis inherent to the aging process. In addition, the procedure is easily performed in the outpatient setting with minimal anesthesia and short downtime and can be coupled with other surgical procedures, such as rhytidectomy, without increased morbidity. Surgeons should offer this type of augmentation to patients seeking a permanent answer to midfacial volume loss and aging in lieu of repeated injections with soft tissue fillers.

SUPPLEMENTARY DATA

Supplementary data related to this article can be found online at http://dx.doi.org/10.1016/j.fsc.2015.01.004.

REFERENCES

1. Plastic surgery statistics report. 2013. Available from the American Society of Plastic Surgeons (ASPS) website: http://www.plasticsurgery.org. Accessed June 18, 2014.
2. Powell N. Proportions of the aesthetic face. New York: Thieme Medical; 1984.
3. Binder WJ. Submalar augmentation: a procedure to enhance rhytidectomy. Ann Plast Surg 1990;24(3):200–12.
4. Binder WJ. Facial rejuvenation and volumization using implants. Facial Plast Surg 2011;27(1):86–97.
5. Quatela VC, Chow J. Synthetic facial implants. Facial Plast Surg Clin North Am 2008;16(1):1–10.
6. Rubin JP, Yaremchuk MJ. Complications and toxicities of implantable biomaterials used in facial reconstructive and aesthetic surgery: a comprehensive review of the literature. Plast Reconstr Surg 1997;100(5):1336–53.
7. Hopping SB, Joshi AS, Tanna N, et al. Volumetric facelift: evaluation of rhytidectomy with alloplastic augmentation. Ann Otol Rhinol Laryngol 2010;119:174–80.

Management of the Midface During Rhytidectomy

Harry Mittelman, MD*, Meir Hershcovitch, MD

KEYWORDS

- Midface rejuvenation • Rhytidectomy
- Multi-vector SMAS (superficial musculoaponeurotic system) lift • Midface lift

KEY POINTS

- The multi-vector high superficial musculoaponeurotic system (SMAS) facelift is a natural extension of a traditional SMAS rhytidectomy.
- There is direct access to the midface with ample opportunity for improvement; the malar fat pad can be addressed directly; the nasolabial grooves and commissure-mandibular grooves can also be improved.
- The extended lower-lid midface lift provides direct access to the midface as well as the ability to provide a direct vertical lift of the midface.

INTRODUCTION

The facial skeleton and bony structures of the face are thought to expand as we age.[1–3] The orbital socket diameter increases in size as we age with particular recession of the inferomedial infraorbital rim.[4] In the midface, the maxilla undergoes retrusion and resorption.[5] The maxillary angle decreased by about 10° between young (aged <30 years) and old (aged >60 years) individuals.[6] Moreover, there is significant development of elastosis of the overlying skin and superficial musculoaponeurotic system (SMAS). There are several telltale signs of aging noted in the midface that can be addressed during rhytidectomy to provide comprehensive and balanced facial rejuvenation. These changes include malar fat pad descent, increasing prominence of the tear trough, an enlarging infraorbicular crescent representing the ptotic inferior orbicularis as well as infraorbital fat,[7] increasing nasolabial grooves, and ptotic and festooning jowls creating a prominent prejowl sulcus.

Various surgical and nonsurgical techniques have been proposed and practiced to rejuvenate the midface. Among the nonsurgical techniques, thermal, radiofrequency, ultrasonic, and various lasers have all been used to refresh the midface. Fillers and injectables including autologous fat transfer have also been used to replace midface volume and mask the descent of anatomic structures. Among surgical treatments, several approaches have been used to rejuvenate and lift the midface, including malar implants, direct lift, multi-vector approach, multi-plane approach, transconjunctival approach, and orbicularis suspension. Many of these techniques, both surgical and nonsurgical, have been used in conjunction with one another and are not mutually exclusive.

One thing remains clear: in order to achieve comprehensive cervicofacial rejuvenation, rhytidectomy remains the gold standard. Tightening and repositioning of redundant skin and the SMAS is paramount to cervicofacial rejuvenation. Unfortunately, too often the midface is neglected

Disclosures: (1) Implantech Board of directors, (2) consultant to Kythera, (3) CosmeSys advisor and investor, (4) advisor to Thermogenics (H. Mittelman); nothing to disclose (M. Hershcovitch).
Mittelman Plastic Surgery Center, 810 Altos Oaks Drive, Los Altos, CA 94085, USA
* Corresponding author.
E-mail address: hmittelman@yahoo.com

leading to suboptimal overall rejuvenation and a continued tired appearance. Posterior SMAS imbrication or plication provides mostly posterior pull and does not adequately address the midface fat pads, nasolabial groove, or commissure-mandibular fold. However, proper midface rejuvenation can be achieved at the same time as cervicofacial rhytidectomy.

TREATMENT GOALS AND PLANNED OUTCOMES

Patients undergoing cervicofacial rhytidectomy nearly uniformly desire comprehensive facial rejuvenation. Midface rejuvenation can easily be improved concurrently with rhytidectomy via a multi-vector, multi-plane approach or an extended lower-lid midface lift. The goals of midface rejuvenation include, but are not limited to, improving the jowl-mandible contour, improving the commissure-mandibular groove, improvement in the nasolabial groove, improving all 4 midface fat pads with repositioning, preserving the temporal hair tuft and posterior hairline, maximizing the cosmetic result, and finally achieving a natural nonoperated appearance. While planning for a surgical procedure, the practitioner must anticipate that different parts of the face and neck require different vectors of pull to achieve an optimal result. The midface in particular requires primarily a vertical lift. The techniques described in this article, multi-vector high SMAS 3-layered facelift with midface lift and extended lower-lid midface lift, achieve all of these goals.

PREOPERATIVE PLANNING AND PREPARATION

The ideal patient is 40 to 60 years old, in good health, without any medical comorbidities or increased bleeding tendencies with significant cervicofacial elastosis, descent of the midface with jowling, prominent jowl-mandibular irregularities, prominent commissure-mandibular grooves, and of course realistic expectations of improvement. Photographic documentation should be obtained preoperatively in the anterior-posterior frame with and without smiling, in a bilateral three-quarter view, and in bilateral side-profile views with particular attention to having each photograph viewing the Frankfort horizontal perpendicularly.

PATIENT POSITIONING

Preoperatively for marking, the authors recommend that patients be seated upright and awake. This *upright* position allows for the proper effects of gravity with respect to the facial architecture as well as certainty that there are no paralytic anesthetics affecting the patients' musculature. Marking is done to demarcate the extent of dissection, the prominence of jowls, and any nasolabial or commissure-mandibular grooves. If an extended lower-lid midface lift is being done, extended lower-lid blepharoplasty incisions should be marked. Very importantly is the marking delineating the directions of the SMAS pull on different areas of the face and neck (**Fig. 1**). This protocol will ideally lead to a more predictable and natural looking result.

PROCEDURAL APPROACH

For the multi-vector high SMAS facelift, perioperatively patients are supine with the endotracheal tube midline or to the left. The tube is secured to the central incisors with a 2-0 silk to allow for movement of the tube on either side of the face. Great care is taken not to allow the endotracheal tube to pull on the lip or the face. The patients' hair is the tied posteriorly and taped out of the surgical field. Patients are then prepped with a half-strength povidone-iodine solution. Towels and sterile tape are then used to further isolate the surgical field.

Firstly, the planned facial incisions were injected with a total of 40 to 60 mL of tumescent solution consisting of a 0.25% bupivacaine hydrochloride (Marcaine), 0.5% lidocaine, and 1:100,000 of epinephrine. The temporal tuft and preauricular, postauricular, and posterior hairline incisions were made with a No. 15 blade; subcutaneous planes were raised in the postauricular area and preauricular area using the same No. 15 blade, and then facelift scissors were used to elevate the same subcutaneous plane anteriorly to a point approximately even with the zygomatic body; but no dissection was made up into the zygomatic body itself. The midface, submandibular, and cervical dissections were made; a 3-0 polypropylene (Prolene) suture was used to vertically raise the SMAS and the anterior cheek perioral area as

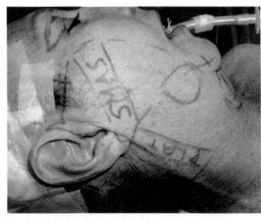

Fig. 1. Marking for multi-vector SMAS lift.

well as the multi-vector SMAS plication (**Figs. 2** and **3**). Softening of the nasolabial and commissure-mandibular grooves as well as elevation of the malar fat pad should be observed.

Several 3-0 Prolene sutures were also used to secure the platysma posteriorly and superiorly to the sternocleidomastoid fascia. The most inferior SMAS suture (3-0 Prolene) vector focuses on improvement of the lower and middle neck. The vector of pull is typically more superior and a little posterior. The most superior SMAS suture, the vectors focus on softening the nasolabial fold and elevating the malar fat pad. That suture's vector of pull is more superior and slightly posterior. The central SMAS sutures focus on improving the submentum, jawline and nasolabial fold. That vector of pull is equally superior and posterior. The elevation of the malar fat pad is considerable during this type of rhytidectomy and care must be taken not to over exaggerate the malar area.

Skin is then redraped and trimmed appropriately, and the skin flaps are closed in the standard fashion. After ensuring adequate hemostasis, the incisions are closed with a 5.0 Prolene suture in a combination of interrupted, running, vertical mattress and horizontal mattress sutures to allow for a tension-free closure (**Figs. 4** and **5**).

An extended lower-lid midface lift may also be used to enhance any facelift or used when doing a lower-lid blepharoplasty. A prominent horizontal lower-lid rhytid is identified, and an incision is marked out and injected with local anesthetic bilaterally. Dissection is carried out deep to the orbicularis muscle bilaterally. Dissection along the lower lid continues in the suborbicularis muscle space, but above the septum orbitale. The dissection of the skin-muscle flap is continued a short distance over the malar prominence depending on that individuals perceived optimal result. Midface mobility allows for suspension of the midface structures

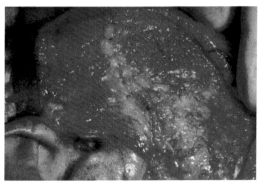

Fig. 3. SMAS suspension in multi-vector facelift with midface suspension.

and inferior orbicularis oculi muscles. The lateral orbicularis is suspended to the orbital rim with horizontal mattress 5-0 Prolene sutures. This suspension allows for focus and suspension of the malar bag. In an attempt to avoid dimpling, the suspension of the inferior orbicularis muscle is accomplished by suturing that muscle to the periosteum 1-4 mm lateral to the lateral orbital rim. An additional suspension of the orbicularis muscle is accomplished 3-6 mm lateral to orbital rim. The two suspensions provide greater assurance that the midface lift elevation will be permanent. The lower lid incisions are closed with interrupted 6-0 prolene laterally and a running 6-0 prolene from the lateral canthus medially. This placement ensures that the suture is placed through the superior portion of the skin-muscle flap to ensure volume before the horizontal mattress is completed on the inferior portion of the skin-muscle flap. The precise placement of these sutures provides smooth contouring of the inferior and superior skin flaps and minimizes the chance of dimpling. The closure is completed by placing interrupted stitches with 6-0 prolene sutures followed by running 6-0 Prolene sutures in the skin bilaterally.

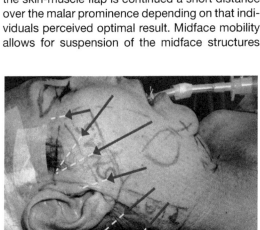

Fig. 2. Vectors of pull for SMAS; medial arrows provide the malar lift.

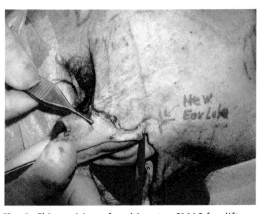

Fig. 4. Skin excision of multi-vector SMAS facelift.

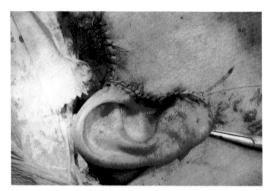

Fig. 5. Closure of multi-vector SMAS facelift.

POTENTIAL COMPLICATIONS AND ADVERSE EVENTS

The multi-vector high SMAS facelift has complications similar to a traditional SMAS plication or imbrication facelift. These complications include, but are not limited to, hematoma, seroma, epidermolysis, hypesthesia, and irregular skin contouring. There is a greater chance of epidermolysis because the blood supply to the skin flap is less compared with a deep-plane technique. Specific midface-related imperfection of the multi-vector high SMAS facelift include too much

elevation of the malar fat pad resulting in too full a malar prominence, usually secondary to too much lift and/or bruising. The fullness of the malar area will typically heal with time. There is always the option to resuspend the midface; however, the authors have never had to do that. In all of the authors' patients, the problem resolved within 2 months.

With regards to the extended lower lid mid-face lift, if there is a lower lid blepharoplasty done concurrently, there is a risk of some lateral rounding. However, in an isolated mid-face lift, the chances are lateral rounding is further diminished because of the suspension of the skin-muscle flap. An adverse effect from the extended lower lid mid-face lift can be irregular skin contouring or dimpling close to the site of the suspension sutures. If dimpling occurs and is cosmetically undesirable, it usually resolves within 2-3 months. If it does not resolve, it can be improved by removing one or both sutures several months after the procedure. A sensation of tightness can be an adverse effect with or without animation in the mid-face, but that resolves within a few weeks if it occurs at all.

POSTPROCEDURAL CARE AND RECOVERY

Care for the multi-vector high SMAS rhytidectomy and midface lift is not dissimilar to traditional

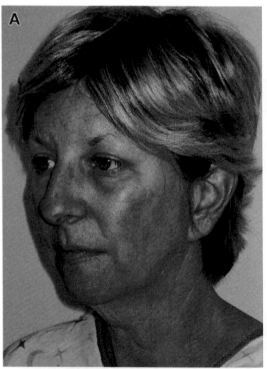

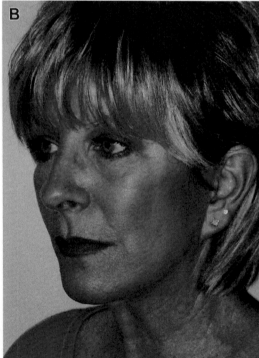

Fig. 6. Preoperative (*A*) and postoperative (*B*) multi-vector SMAS facelift combined with chin-prejowl implant and rhinoplasty.

care after a rhytidectomy. All patients receive anti-staphylococcal antibiotics for 5 days postoperatively. The authors recommend follow-up visits to the office the day after surgery for the first postoperative visit and dressing change. On the fourth or fifth day, the first set of sutures are removed. Additional sutures are removed 1 week postoperatively, and all sutures are usually

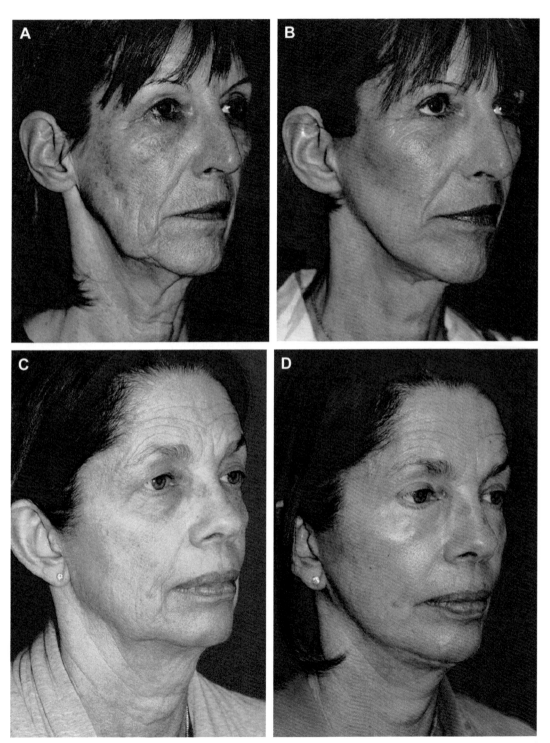

Fig. 7. Preoperative (*A, C*) and postoperative (*B, D*) extended lower-lid midface lift with concurrent face-neck lift and vertical neck lift.

removed between 10 days to 2 weeks postoperatively. The authors also recommends sleeping with the head of the bed elevated for 2 weeks as well as restriction of rotational movement of the head and neck for 6 weeks. The patient needs to clean the crusting of the incisions several times a day until sutures are removed. Pain control is achieved with acetaminophen-hydrocodone; however, often extra-strength acetaminophen is all that is needed.

Postoperative care following an extended lower-lid midface lift is similar to that of a blepharoplasty. Skin sutures are typically removed in a staged fashion between 3 and 7 days after surgery. The authors recommend that ice packs should be applied to the eyes shortly after surgery. Ice packs should be applied in 20-minute intervals (20 minutes on, 20 minutes off) while awake for the first 2 to 3 days after surgery. It is recommended that there is no direct contact between ice and the incision; use a washcloth or gauze as a buffer instead. The incisions should be cleaned with a gauze pad or cotton tips using tepid water to remove any crusts that may form. A thin layer of the hydrophilic ointment to the suture line 3 times a day also aids in this task. Pain control is typically achieved with extra-strength acetaminophen.

RESULTS AND CONCLUSION

Different parts of the face and neck require a different vector of pull for optimal results. Both the multi-vector high SMAS facelift and extended lower-lid midface lift adequately address the midface during rhytidectomy. The most medial portion of the dissection with SMAS plication results in a primarily vertical lift of the malar fat pad in a multi-vector high SMAS facelift. In a typical deep plane, SMAS facelift, or as a stand alone

procedure, the midface may be addressed with an extended lower-lid midface lift. This procedure allows for direct access to the midface and a direct superior and slightly posterior pull of the midface fat pads. The goals of both of these procedures are to improve the position of the midface fat pads. These procedures can be an adjunct to traditional rhytidectomy and allow for comprehensive facial rejuvenation. Preoperative and postoperative examples of the multi-vector high SMAS facelift and extended lower-lid midface lift are shown in **Figs. 6** and **7**, respectively.

REFERENCES

1. Hellman M. Changes in the human face brought about by development. Int J Orthod 1927;13:475.
2. Todd TW. Thickness of the white male cranium. Anat Rec 1924;27:245.
3. Garn SM, Rohmann CG, Wagner B, et al. Continuing bone growth during adult life: a general phenomenon. Am J Phys Anthropol 1967;26:313.
4. Kahn DM, Shaw RB Jr. Aging of the bony orbit: a three-dimensional computed tomographic study. Aesthet Surg J 2008;28:258–64.
5. Pessa JE. An algorithm of facial aging: verification of Lambros's theory by three-dimensional stereolithography, with reference to the pathogenesis of midfacial aging, scleral show, and the lateral suborbital trough deformity. Plast Reconstr Surg 2000;106:479–88.
6. Mendelson BC, Hartley W, Scott M, et al. Age-related changes of the orbit and midcheek and the implications for facial rejuvenation. Aesthetic Plast Surg 2007;31:419–23.
7. Furnas DW. Festoons of orbicularis muscle as a cause of baggy eyelids. Plast Reconstr Surg 1978; 61:540–6.

Endoscopic Midfacial Rejuvenation

Robert D. Engle, MD[a], Taylor R. Pollei, MD[b,c], Edwin F. Williams III, MD[b,c],*

KEYWORDS

• Facial rejuvenation • Subperiosteal midface lift • Rhytidectomy • Endoscopic midface lift

KEY POINTS

• The midface and lower lid aging processes are highly interdependent, and attempts at rejuvenation must address both simultaneously.
• The aging process results from soft tissue volume loss, vertical descent of soft tissue, loss of bony projection, and laxity of the overlying skin. Each component must be considered in developing a strategy for rejuvenation.
• Endoscopic subperiosteal lift allows for an ideal vector of suspension, but has limited effect on the nasolabial fold.
• Endoscopic malar lift specifically addresses the nasolabial fold.

INTRODUCTION

Despite the increasing popularity of surgical facial rejuvenation during the 20th century, surgical treatment of the midface was largely ignored. The process of midfacial aging was poorly understood and misinterpreted. To address the midface, patients underwent blepharoplasty with skin and fat resection without addressing the cheek/midface complex, which often exacerbated the aged appearance.

In 1976, the description of the superficial musculoaponeurotic system (SMAS) by Mitz and Peyronie greatly advanced the understanding of midface anatomy.[1] Hamra advanced surgical techniques with sub-SMAS dissection, advocating deep plane and composite lifting of the midface.[2] In the following years, the subperiosteal approach to the upper face was described, along with extended access to the midface via bicoronal incision.[3] In 1994, Ramirez pioneered and popularized the endoscopic midface lift with subperiosteal dissection over the malar eminence and inferior orbital rim via temporal and intraoral approaches, providing effective elevation of the junction between the lower lid and midface.[4] Further, this approach avoided dissection through the preseptal orbicularis oculi.

The senior author has employed the endoscopic subperiosteal approach to the midface since 1995. In the initial 75 cases, gingivobuccal sulcus incisions were utilized to assist with dissection, but these were ultimately abandoned in favor of dissection via temporal incisions alone. The endoscopic midface lift was performed in conjunction with endoscopic brow lift to prevent redundancy of temporal skin. When indicated, blepharoplasty was performed in the same operative setting with skin pinch and transconjunctival fat excision, thus preventing disruption of the middle lamella and minimizing risks of lower lid malposition.

One key concept is that the aging and subsequent rejuvenation of the midface and lower eyelid do not occur in isolation. The aging effects on the

Financial Disclosure and Conflict of Interest: None.
[a] Division of Otolaryngology and Head-Neck Surgery, Department of Surgery, Albany Medical College, 50 New Scotland Avenue, 4th Floor, Albany, NY 12209, USA; [b] Division of Otolaryngology and Head-Neck Surgery, Department of Surgery, Albany Medical College, Albany, NY 12209, USA; [c] Department of Facial Plastic and Reconstructive Surgery, Williams Center for Excellence, 1072 Troy Schenectady Road, Latham, NY 12110, USA
* Corresponding author. Williams Center for Excellence, 1072 Troy Schenectady Road, Latham, NY 12110.
E-mail address: edwilliams@nelasersurg.com

lower lid and lower face are more appreciated now than ever before. Elevation of the midfacial soft tissues results in shortening of the lower lid with additional soft tissue support, while simultaneously tightening the orbicularis oculi sling with the slight horizontal vector of lifting. Further, this elevation in the midface may improve soft tissue crowding in the jowl area. Despite successful repositioning of the malar fat pad, the nasolabial fold usually is not significantly effaced by this technique. This will be further discussed, but ultimately this remains a limitation that proponents of this approach are willing to accept in exchange for the safety and efficacy of this procedure.

Midfacial aging is multifactorial, with the 4 greatest contributors being soft tissue volume loss, soft tissue ptosis, bony remodeling with decreased projection, and overlying skin changes. Attempts at rejuvenation must be individualized to each patient, with consideration given to each component of midfacial aging. Frequently, patient preference dictates initial intervention with volume restoration through fillers. Once this is not adequate or appropriate to achieve the desired result, surgical intervention is directed to address the patient's greatest deficiencies within the midface. The techniques described herein represent a single modality, while most commonly multiple modalities are combined to create the best possible aesthetic result. Further, the surgical intervention can be thought of as an adjustment of the patient's baseline, from which fillers and resurfacing techniques can be used to refine and maintain the rejuvenation. The described technique is frequently combined with an endoscopic brow lift procedure in order to avoid bunching of excess skin and soft tissue at the lateral canthus and temporal region. For patients in whom a brow lift is not indicated, other options exist for correction of soft tissue ptosis. Although not ideal for the midface, the deep plane facelift originally described by Hamra will most closely approximate the optimal vector of suspension that is achieved in endoscopic techniques.

Innumerable techniques have been described in efforts to attain adequate rejuvenation of the midface while maximizing consistency in results and avoiding morbidity. Here is presented a strong bias toward the endoscopic subperiosteal midface lift over other described techniques. This bias is wrought on the basis of extensive trauma experience in accessing the midface and the senior author's experience of over 1200 cases and patient follow-up spanning nearly 20 years. The authors believe the described technique to be safe, effective, and well within the abilities of most practitioners of facial plastic surgery. The endoscopic malar fat pad lift is presented as an alternative technique for surgical rejuvenation of the midface, with emphasis on improvement of the nasolabial fold.

ANATOMY

A thorough understanding of midfacial anatomy is necessary in any attempt at midfacial rejuvenation. The boundaries of the midface are somewhat indistinct and have been defined with variability throughout the literature. The authors find it most advantageous to define the midface as an inverted triangle with the apex at the nasolabial fold. The lateral border is a line connecting this apex to the lateral canthus, and the medial border is a line connecting the apex along the nasolabial fold to the medial canthus. Classically, the superior limit of the midface has been defined as a horizontal line at the inferior orbital rim. In recent years, the concept of the lower lid and the midface as a single interrelated unit has been popularized. The impact of attempts at midfacial rejuvenation on the lower lid cannot be overstated, and thus the authors consider the superior border of the midface to be the inferior border of the lower lid tarsal plate. This supports the need to address the orbicularis oculi sling in midfacial rejuvenation.

The 3-dimensional volume and contours of the midface are best understood by their individual volumetric contributors. The superficial volumetric contributors are the malar fat pad and superficial orbital fat. The middle adipose layer of the midface consists of the suborbicularis oculi fat (SOOF) and medial deep cheek fat. The deep adipose layer of consists of the medial and lateral deep cheek fat compartments (**Fig. 1**).[5]

The malar fat pad represents the thickening of the subcutaneous fat overlying the maxilla. This triangular volume is superficial to the SMAS and creates much of the prezygomatic convexity associated with the youthful midface. Dissections by Rohrich and Pessa illustrate that the malar fat pad is in fact divided into distinct compartments: nasolabial, medial, middle cheek, and lateral temporal cheek. These compartments are separated by condensations of the superficial fascia and with dense dermal attachments.[5] Some of these facial condensations are thought to be the retaining ligaments of the face and may contain perforating vessels.[6]

The subcutaneous orbital fat is also divided into 3 compartments: superior, inferior, and lateral. The inferior and lateral compartments must be considered when addressing the aging midface. The inferior compartment is bounded superiorly by the inferior border of the tarsus, and inferiorly by the orbicularis retaining ligament (ORL), with these 2 structures joining at the medial and lateral canthi. The lateral orbital fat compartment is bounded

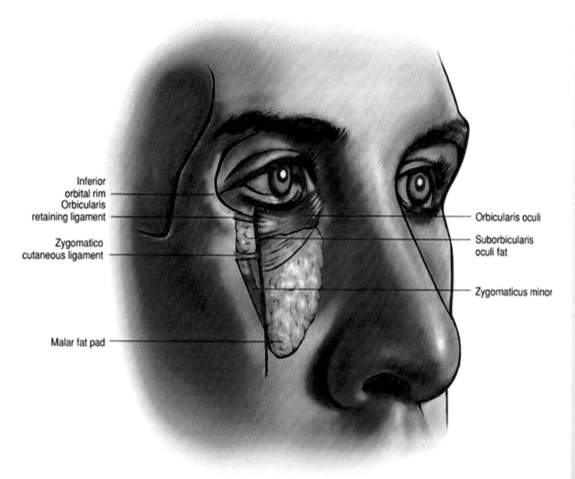

Inferior orbital rim
Orbicularis retaining ligament
Zygomatico cutaneous ligament
Malar fat pad
Orbicularis oculi
Suborbicularis oculi fat
Zygomaticus minor

Fig. 1. Anatomy of the midface: musculature, fat pads, and retaining ligaments. (*From* Yeh CC, Williams EF. Long-term results of autologous periorbital lipotransfer. Arch Facial Plast Surg 2011;13(4):252–58; with permission.)

superiorly by the inferior temporal septum and inferiorly by the superior cheek septum. Notably, the zygomaticus major muscle is adherent to the deep surface of this compartment.[5]

The SOOF represents a much smaller volume of the midface relative to the malar fat pad, but it can play a dramatic role in the appearance of the midface. The SOOF lies inferior to the inferior orbital rim, deep to the orbicularis oculi, superficial to the preperiosteal layer. It is divided into 2 distinct compartments, with the medial compartment existing between the medial limbus and lateral canthus, and the lateral compartment between the lateral canthus to the temporal fat pad. The inferior boundary of the SOOF is the tear trough. Nasal to the medial compartment of the SOOF is the medial deep cheek fat.[7]

The nasolabial compartment of the malar fat lies anterior to the medial deep cheek fat. It is bounded superiorly by the ORL and anteriorly by the nasolabial fold; it overlaps the jowl fat compartment

inferiorly. The lower border of zygomaticus major is adherent to the inferior portion of this compartment.[5] The relative volume of this compartment and the lack of volume loss in aging are major determinants in the prominence of the nasolabial fold. The nasolabial fold itself represents dense fibrous connections between the superficial muscles of facial expression and the overlying dermis. Contraction of these muscles works to deepen the fold over time.[8] To achieve improvement in the nasolabial fold, the relative position of the superficial muscles of facial expression and the nasolabial fat compartment must be altered. The subperiosteal midface lift results in suspension of both of these structures en masse, and therefore cannot be expected to address the nasolabial fold. The endoscopic malar fat pad lift is designed to specifically address this portion of the midface anatomy.[9]

The jowl fat compartment is inferior and deep to the nasolabial fat. It is adherent to the depressor anguli oris and bounded medially by the lip depressor musculature.[5] Similar maintenance of volume in this compartment despite aging and descent results in prominence of the prejowl sulcus.

Midfacial soft tissue ptosis has effects beyond simple vertical descent. Typically this has the most pronounced impact through displacement of the malar fat pad from the well-supported premalar region to the poorly supported infrazygomatic region. This is compounded by malar bone regression and elongation of the bony orbit with age.[10]

The anatomic hallmark of all temporal approaches to the midface is the specific position of the temporal branch(es) of the facial nerve. The surface landmark most commonly referenced is the Pitanguy line, from 0.5 cm below the tragus to 1.5 cm above the lateral brow.[11] Alternatively, a line drawn from the bottom of the ear lobe to the midpoint between the superior border of the tragus and the lateral canthus can approximate the position of the temporal branch.[12] This nerve exits the superior pole of the parotid gland at the inferior border of the zygoma, at which point it continues anterosuperiorly over the arch and is densely adherent to the periosteum. Once above the arch, the nerve enters the superficial temporal fat pad and joins the undersurface of the superficial temporal fascia or temporoparietal fascia (TPF). This is the continuation of the SMAS layer above the zygomatic arch. Deep to this layer is the deep temporal fascia, which in turn divides into superficial and deep layers around the intermediate temporal fat pad. The superficial layer of the deep temporal fascia inserts on the superolateral zygomatic periosteum, while the deep layer of the deep temporal fascia inserts superomedially. Incision and elevation of the zygomatic periosteum at or deep to the insertion of the superficial layer of the deep temporal fascia will provide protection of the temporal branches of the facial nerve.

SUBPERIOSTEAL MIDFACE LIFT
Procedure

The temporal approach subperiosteal midface lift is typically performed in conjunction with an endoscopic brow lift procedure. This allows for rejuvenation of the entire upper two-thirds of the face with a single consolidated surgical technique, while simultaneously avoiding bunching of excess skin at the lateral canthus and temporal region. This procedure is described in detail elsewhere,[13] so here is presented the concise procedure with key points. As described, it may be performed under either monitored anesthesia care with intravenous sedation or general anesthesia. Five standard endoscopic brow lift incisions are marked, including midline, parasagittal at the lateral canthus, and about 1 cm

posterior and parallel to the temporal hairline. The hair is secured with paper tape, and local anesthetic with epinephrine is infiltrated at the incision sites and subperiosteally along the orbital rim. The midline and medial incisions are made through periosteum, and an endoscopic brow lift is performed, including release of the arcus marginalis, thinning of the currugator and procerus musculature, and the conjoined tendon of the superior temporal line. At the lateral (temporal) incisions, dissection is performed down to the superficial layer of the deep temporal fascia. This plane is opened bluntly across the entire temporal region and down to the zygomatic arch. In the region of the Pitanguy line, one or more prominent perforating veins will be encountered. These have been shown to indicate position of the temporal branch in the lateral soft tissues, with an accuracy of plus or minus 2 mm. Initially, these vessels were ligated for exposure and mobility, but in time it was realized that these veins could be skeletonized and preserved, allowing both adequate access to the midface, and mobility of the soft tissues for suspension. Preservation of these vessels anecdotally diminished postoperative edema, which has been a criticism of the subperiosteal dissection technique.[9] In addition, ligation of these vessels was found to result in an unfavorable increased prominence of superficial lateral orbital veins. Preservation of a 1 cm cuff of soft tissue surrounding the lateral canthus has been shown to successfully prevent lateral canthus displacement with this procedure.[14] The conjoint temporalis tendon is divided sharply, and a sharp incision is made onto the periosteum of the zygoma with utmost care to remain deep to the superficial temporal fasical (TPF). This ensures protection of the temporal branch of the facial nerve.

One key distinction is that the endoscopic designation of these procedures has become somewhat of a misnomer. The described approaches were initially performed using rigid telescopes, but the senior author rapidly moved away from endoscopic visualization to direct visualization through incisions of the same size. A converse retractor and headlight were found to provide an excellent optical cavity and visualization for dissection of the upper face and temporal region. As subperiosteal dissection progresses over the anterior zygoma and onto the maxilla, dissection is guided by the surgeon's nondominant hand on the skin rather than via direct visualization. Knowledge of the infraorbital neurovascular bundle location is critical for safe dissection at this point of the procedure. Elevation progresses over the maxilla and inferior orbital rim using a curved dissector while protecting the orbit and infraorbital nerve with the nondominant hand. Gingivobuccal incision remains an option for additional access to the maxilla and direct visualization of the infraorbital nerve. The senior author moved away from this technique early in his experience, finding it unnecessary with increased morbidity and an increased infection rate, incisional discomfort, and prolonged edema. Inferior to the zygomatic arch, 1 cm of masseteric fascia is dissected bluntly, allowing release of the zygomaticus major but avoiding release of masseter itself. This dissection pocket is bluntly connected to the subperiosteal dissection of the maxilla. This provides complete release of the midfacial soft tissues. Suspension is first performed at the medial browlift incision to address the brow and temporal regions and prevent bunching around the lateral canthus. Unilateral midfacial suspension is then achieved with a single suture, passed through the malar fat pad and adjacent zygomaticus major and suspended to the deep temporal fascia. Other authors have advocated for multiple suture suspension[12] or absorbable fixation devices such as the Endotine (MicroAire, Charlottesville, Virginia).[15] However, the senior author has not encountered the need for suspension beyond a single, properly placed suture. Regardless of the suspension technique, initially both sides should be suspended simultaneously to ensure symmetry of the lift. Once the surgeon has gained adequate experience, each side may be completed independently with excellent outcomes.

Complications

Of all complications associated with the subperiosteal midface lift, motor nerve injury is the most feared. In a previous 5-year review of the senior author's outcomes with this technique in 325 patients, 3 patients developed temporary frontal branch weakness, and 1 patient developed buccal distribution weakness. All resolved completely within 6 months.[16] In the same study, 1 patient experienced permanent infraorbital anesthesia, and 2 patients experienced malar subperiosteal abscesses requiring incision and drainage. One of these patients eventually required an alloplastic implant to correct the resultant volume loss. Notably, both abscesses occurred with the additional intraoral incision. Revision rates for this technique are reported at less than 1%.[17] Hematoma rates are similarly reported at less than 1%, and may be more difficult to identify than typical rhytidectomy hematoma due to the thickness of the flap. Excessive swelling of the midface and ecchymoses at the gingivobuccal sulcus are generally indicative of hematoma. The thickness and robust blood supply of the flap generally prevent flap ischemia in the case of hematoma.[12]

ENDOSCOPIC MALAR FAT LIFT

This procedure is performed in isolation or immediately prior to an endoscopic browlift. Access is provided through an incision camouflaged by the crow's foot rhytids at the lateral canthus. Dissection is performed under the orbicularis oculi until the malar attachment of zygomaticus major is identified. Dissection progresses along the superficial surface of zygomaticus major and its SMAS investment, toward the commissura labiorum and ending at the nasolabial fold. Once the malar fat is identified, the zygomatic ligaments superior and lateral to this structure are divided. A suture is passed through the deep aspect of the malar fat and suspended to the lateral orbital rim periosteum if performed in isolation, or the deep temporal fascia if performed with browplasty.[9]

This procedure specifically addresses the appearance of the nasolabial fold by altering the relationship of the nasolabial compartment of the malar fat to the underlying muscles of facial expression. It will simultaneously reposition malar fat over the bony malar eminence and can be expected to restore midfacial projection and volume. In contrast to the subperiosteal midface lift, the malar fat pad lift will not produce upturning of the oral commissure.

Complications

The most common issue following endoscopic malar fat pad lift is edema around the incision, adjacent to the lateral canthus. This may remain up to 6 weeks postoperatively, but patient concerns are typically only present in the first 10 to 14 days. Edema and redundancy may be minimized by concomitant endoscopic brow lift. In cases of severe malar wasting, dimpling of the skin may result from the suspension suture closely affecting fibrous dermal attachments. This should be recognized as a contraindication to this type of procedure.[9] A review of 472 cases of malar suspension showed a revision rate of less than 3%, relating to suboptimal aesthetic results, and concurrent procedures were common at the time of revision. Minor complications occurred in about 1% of patients, with no reported hematoma or infection.[18]

DISCUSSION

The endoscopic subperiosteal midface lift is a powerful tool for addressing the aging midface (**Figs. 2** and **3**). The endoscopic malar fat lift represents an excellent option for patients whose primary concern is the appearance of the nasolabial fold. Both endoscopic approaches are appealing for patients, because they minimize/camouflage incisions and carry the notion of a minimally invasive surgical technique. Endoscopic techniques also appeal to surgeons by providing favorable aesthetic results with a minimum of inherent risk and patient

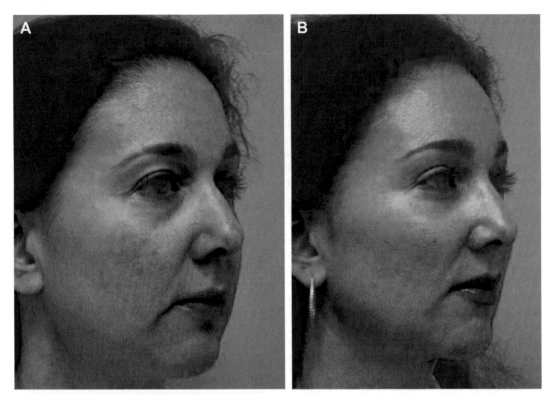

Fig. 2. (A) Preoperative midface lift with browlift and upper eyelid blepharoplasty. (B) Postoperative midface lift with browlift and upper eyelid blepharoplasty.

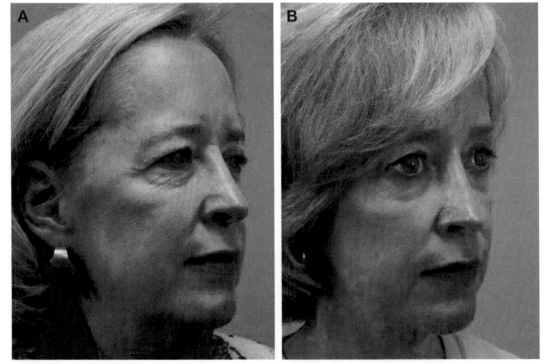

Fig. 3. (A) Preoperative midface lift with facelift, browlift, and upper eyelid blepharoplasty. (B) Postoperative midface lift with facelift, browlift, and upper eyelid blepharoplasty.

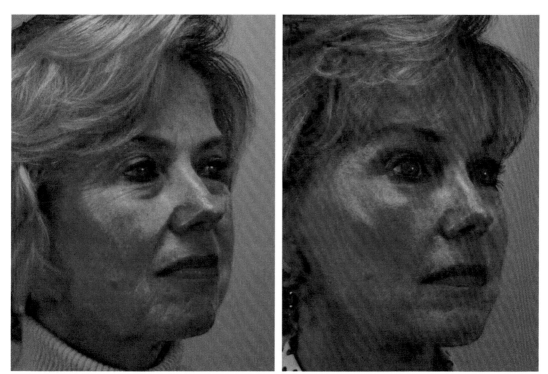

Fig. 4. (*A*) Preoperative midface lift with facelift, full face 35% TCA peel, and upper and lower blepharoplasty in addition to bilateral midface/lower orbit autologous lipotransfer. (*B*) Postoperative midface lift with facelift, full face 35% TCA peel, and upper and lower blepharoplasty in addition to bilateral midface/lower orbit autologous lipotransfer.

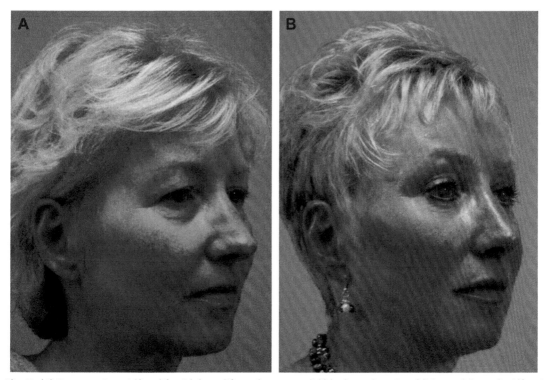

Fig. 5. (*A*) Preoperative midface lift with browlift, and upper eyelid blepharoplasty in addition to bilateral midface/lower orbit autologous lipotransfer. (*B*) Postoperative midface lift with browlift, and upper eyelid blepharoplasty in addition to bilateral midface/lower orbit autologous lipotransfer.

morbidity, and the directed dissection techniques make efficient use of the surgeon's time. The greatest difficulty comes in selecting patients for these procedures and how to blend the surgical correction with the proper adjunctive treatments (eg, skeletal augmentation, resurfacing, volumization) to provide the patient with the optimal aesthetic outcome. As a result, it is the authors' experience that combining the midface lift with autologous lipotransfer provides improved results when compared with midface lift alone (**Figs. 4** and **5**).

REFERENCES

1. Mitz V, Peyronie M. The superficial musculo-aponeurotic system (SMAS) in the parotid and cheek area. Plast Reconstr Surg 1976;58:80–8.

2. Hamra ST. The deep-plane rhytidectomy. Plast Reconstr Surg 1990;86:53–61 [discussion: 62–3].

3. Psillakis JM, Rumley TO, Camargos A. Subperiosteal approach as an improved concept for correction of the aging face. Plast Reconstr Surg 1988;82:383–94.

4. Ramirez OM. Endoscopic full facelift. Aesthetic Plast Surg 1994;18:363–71.

5. Rohrich RJ, Pessa JE. The fat compartments of the face: anatomy and clinical implications for cosmetic surgery. Plast Reconstr Surg 2007;119:2219–27 [discussion: 2228–31].

6. Rohrich RJ, Pessa JE. The retaining system of the face: histologic evaluation of the septal boundaries of the subcutaneous fat compartments. Plast Reconstr Surg 2008;121:1804–9.

7. Rohrich RJ, Arbique GM, Wong C, et al. The anatomy of suborbicularis fat: implications for periorbital rejuvenation. Plast Reconstr Surg 2009;124:946–51.

8. Rubin LR. The anatomy of the nasolabial fold: the keystone of the smiling mechanism. Plast Reconstr Surg 1999;103:687–91 [discussion: 692–84].

9. Freeman MS. Endoscopic techniques for rejuvenation of the midface. Facial Plast Surg Clin North Am 2005;13:141–55.

10. Shaw RB Jr, Katzel EB, Koltz PF, et al. Aging of the facial skeleton: aesthetic implications and rejuvenation strategies. Plast Reconstr Surg 2011;127:374–83.

11. Pitanguy I, Ramos AS. The frontal branch of the facial nerve: the importance of its variations in face lifting. Plast Reconstr Surg 1966;38:352–6.

12. Quatela VC, Azzi JP, Antunes MB. Endoscopic-assisted facelifting. Facial Plast Surg 2014;30:413–21.

13. Williams EF, Lam SM. Comprehensive facial rejuvenation: a practical and systematic guide to surgical management of the aging face. Philadelphia: Lippincott Williams & Wilkins; 2004.

14. Kolstad CK, Quatela VC. A quantitative analysis of lateral canthal position following endoscopic forehead-midface-lift surgery. JAMA Facial Plast Surg 2013;15:352–7.

15. Saltz R, Ohana B. Thirteen years of experience with the endoscopic midface lift. Aesthet Surg J 2012;32:927–36.

16. Williams EF 3rd, Vargas H, Dahiya R, et al. Midfacial rejuvenation via a minimal-incision brow-lift approach: critical evaluation of a 5-year experience. Arch Facial Plast Surg 2003;5:470–8.

17. Quatela VC, Marotta JC. Pitfalls of midface surgery. Facial Plast Surg Clin North Am 2005;13:401–9.

18. de la Torre JI, Rosenberg LZ, De Cordier BC, et al. Clinical analysis of malar fat pad re-elevation. Ann Plast Surg 2003;50:244–8 [discussion: 248].

Transpalpebral Midface Lift

Anthony P. Sclafani, MD[a,b,*], Gregory Dibelius, MD[a]

KEYWORDS

- Aging face • Facial rejuvenation • Midface • Facelift • Transpalpebral • Blepharoplasty

KEY POINTS

- Midface rejuvenation procedures have evolved from laterally based rhytidectomy techniques to centrofacial approaches with more vertical vectors of elevation.
- Volume loss and remodeling of the maxillofacial skeleton should be addressed with various augmentation procedures.
- Patients with prominent globe/negative vectors or previous lower eyelid surgery are at increased risk for postoperative lid malposition.
- Lateral canthal support procedures range from simple midface elevation and suspension to formal canthotomy/cantholysis with lateral canthal reconstruction; selecting the appropriate technique should be guided by individual patient concerns and surgeon experience and skill.
- The tear trough and nasolabial fold can be difficult areas to correct surgically; fillers, autologous free fat or superficial musculoaponeurotic system (SMAS) grafts, or allografts can be transferred to the tear trough area or nasolabial folds.

 A video of transpalpebral midface rejuvenation accompanies this article at http://www. facialplastic.theclinics.com/

The midface is an important facial aesthetic sub-unit and may exhibit many of the telltale signs of aging. Aging occurs within each of the anatomic layers of the midface, with changes visible as early as the third decade. Descent of atrophic skin and attenuation of orbicularis musculature are often associated with pseudoherniation of orbital fat, outwardly transforming the smooth concavity of the eyelid-cheek junction into a double convexity. Tarsoligamentous laxity leads to visible length-ening of the lower lid, and the eye assumes a rounded shape with a negative canthal tilt. Crow's-feet form at the superolateral boundary of the midface. Soft tissues over the malar eminence, in particular the subcutaneous malar fat pad and midface retaining ligaments, become ptotic and descend, reducing malar prominence and skeletonizing the inferior orbital rim, creating a hollowed appearance. Malar bags and festoons manifest within the superficial layers. A nasojugal trough becomes apparent medially, resulting in the so-called tear trough deformity. The depen-dent region of the nasolabial crease becomes burdened with ptotic superolateral soft tissues, giving rise to a hooded appearance and a deep-ening of the fold. Volume loss has been increas-ingly appreciated as an important part of the aging process as well progressive remodeling of the maxillofacial skeleton. The skin of the face un-dergoes typical actinic processes. The sum of these changes leads to the characteristically tired appearance associated with age, with the overall

Disclosures: The authors have no relevant disclosures.
[a] Department of Otolaryngology-Head and Neck Surgery, New York Eye and Ear Infirmary of Mount Sinai, 310 East 14th Street, New York, NY 10003, USA; [b] Department of Otolaryngology- Head and Neck Surgery, Icahn School of Medicine at Mount Sinai, 310 East 14th Street, New York, NY 10003, USA
* Corresponding author. Department of Otolaryngology- Head and Neck Surgery, Icahn School of Medicine at Mount Sinai, 310 East 14th Street, New York, NY 10003.
E-mail address: asclafani@nyee.edu

Facial Plast Surg Clin N Am 23 (2015) 209–219
http://dx.doi.org/10.1016/j.fsc.2015.01.007
1064-7406/15/$ – see front matter © 2015 Elsevier Inc. All rights reserved.

loss of the heart-shaped face of youth. A thorough understanding of the anatomy of the midface and its age-associated pathophysiology is essential to the safe and effective performance of midface rejuvenation.

ANATOMY AND PATHOPHYSIOLOGY

Surgical midface anatomy is complex. Skin, various fat pads, the SMAS, mimetic musculature, neurovascular structures, retaining ligaments, and periosteum overlie the facial skeleton in a layered fashion. Critical structures pertaining to transpalpebral facelift techniques include the lower lid skin, orbital septum, lateral canthal tendon, orbicularis oculi muscle, suborbicularis oculi fat (SOOF) and malar fat pads, and zygomatic and orbicularis retaining ligaments.

The anatomy of the orbicularis oculi is central to discussion of transpalpebral techniques. It is a facial mimetic muscle and an integral part of the SMAS, functioning as the ocular sphincter. It is composed of a central pars palpebralis and a peripheral pars orbitalis, and, together with the lower eyelid skin, comprises the anterior lamellae of the eyelid. Its orbital part underlies the subcutaneous malar fat pad as it radiates inferiorly across the lid-cheek junction, whereas the SOOF pad lies deep to the muscle and generates a natural glide plane that allows the muscle to move independently over the underlying periosteum and origins of the lip elevator muscles. This plane has been described in thoughtful anatomic study as the prezygomatic space.[1] The orbicularis retaining ligament attaches the deep aspect of the orbicularis muscle to the inferolateral orbital rim periosteum, forming the superior boundary of the prezygomatic space and separating it from the preseptal space of the lower eyelid. This ligament has also been interpreted as an orbitomalar ligament, inserting into the dermis through the muscle body; regardless, release or elevation of this ligament is fundamental to achieving satisfactory elevation of deep midface tissues. Laterally, this ligament expands and joins the lateral orbital thickening, which overlies the bony inferolateral orbital rim and represents a confluence of the major superficial and deep fascias of the lateral orbital and temporal regions. Inferiorly, zygomatico-cutaneous ligaments arise between the zygomaticus muscles to fix the malar fat pad and cheek skin to zygomatic eminence. These are also important retaining ligaments of the midface that must be released to elevate deep tissues and define the inferior extent of the prezygomatic space (discussed previously). The lateral canthal tendon is a critical support structure that anchors the lateral canthus to the bony orbit

and is contiguous with the superficial fascial component that joins the lateral orbital thickening.[2] It defines the lateral canthus of the eye and damage to or improper reconstruction of the lateral canthal tendon can lead to significant cosmetic deformity. Inferiorly, the nasolabial fold represents an area of confluence of tissues at the lower border of the midface, where fasciofibrous connections of the SMAS and mimetic musculature join with the dermis.

TRANSPALPEBRAL APPROACHES

Hester and colleagues are credited with the introduction of the skin-muscle flap approach to the midface in 1996.[3–6] Their technique demonstrated the importance of proactive lower lid support and showed that multiple points of reliable suture fixation are essential to achieving stable fixation. They also emphasized conservative skin resection and defined the major tenets of the transblepharoplasty midface approaches. In 1999, Gunter and Hackney modified this procedure to avoid requisite lateral canthoplasty, pioneering a different approach the management of the lateral canthus.[6]

Access to the midface is typically subciliary, as in Hester and colleagues' original technique, or transconjunctival. The former offers the ability to perform conservative skin and muscle resection and affords wider exposure to the midface but carries a theoretic risk of microdenervation of the pretarsal orbicularis muscle. The latter preserves orbicularis innervation and minimizes septal manipulation that may lead to contracture and lid retraction but has more limited exposure (which may be improved by adding a canthotomy).[7] Patients with significant malar bags or festoons may benefit from a traditional skin-muscle flap technique, because these superficial deformities are unlikely to be corrected via a transconjunctival approach.[8]

KEY CONSIDERATIONS IN LOWER BLEPHAROPLASTY

Preoperative assessment should include an ophthalmic history and evaluation. Dry eyes, prior procedures, glaucoma, and inflammatory conditions should be noted. Patients should be counseled that patients prone to dry eyes tend to have worsening of symptoms in the postoperative period and the need for ocular lubricants should be discussed. Surgery may not be appropriate for some of these patients. Of critical importance to aesthetic surgeons and patients is avoiding malposition of the lower lid and lateral canthus. Patients with prominent globe or negative vector, in whom the plane of the cornea is anterior to the plane of the bony orbital rim, as well those who have undergone lower lid surgery are at increased risk for postoperative lid malposition. Preoperative or intraoperative distraction and snap tests should be performed to assess lid laxity and further discern the need for conservative anterior lamella resection or anticipated need for lower lid support.

Pseudoherniation of orbital fat is well known to give rise to contour irregularities of the lower eyelid. In midface surgery, this particular deformity requires additional consideration and must be dealt with in a thoughtful manner. Conservative resection of lower lid fat compartments can be performed during a transblepharoplasty midface lift, with limited resection of fat, particularly in the nasal and midfat compartments. Temporal fat tends to be more forgiving and may be excised more aggressively, which is done routinely by some surgeons.[9,10] The need for conservative resection of fat should be carefully assessed preoperatively and intraoperatively once the flap is elevated. After release of the arcus marginalis, infraorbital fat can be used to redrape the skeletonized inferior orbital rim and fill in the nasojugal trough.[11,12] Elevation of the midface soft tissues with arcus marginalis release may provide adequate correction of those irregularities preoperatively attributed to pseudoherniation, and over-aggressive fat excision, therefore, may lead to lower lid complications.

TECHNIQUE

The specific techniques described represent those preferred by the senior author (APS).[13,14] These described procedures nonetheless illustrates the essential techniques of transpalpebral midface rejuvenation (Video 1).

The transpalpebral midface lift can be performed under intravenous sedation or general anesthesia and with the subciliary approach in carefully selected patients, even under local anesthesia. Careful regional nerve blockade should be applied, and local anesthesia can be infiltrated along planned incision lines.

Both subciliary and transconjunctival incisions can be used to perform a transpalpebral midface lift, depending on the anticipated extent of lower lid skin resection. Preoperative evaluation of lower lid laxity with snap and distraction tests aids in this determination.

In patients who do not have significant lower lid skin redundancy, a transconjunctival incision with canthotomy and cantholysis is performed. A small incision is made from the lateral canthus extending to a point 4 to 6 mm laterally within an existing crow's-feet rhytid. A straight clamp is introduced straddling the lateral canthal conjunctiva and used to crush the soft tissue to limit bleeding, and the incision is carried down to bone using electrocautery. Cantholysis is carried out using curved Stevens scissors, directed inferiorly to divide the inferior limb of the lateral canthal tendon.

The transconjunctival incision is then made approximately 3 mm below the inferior tarsal border and is carried laterally to join the canthotomy incision. Dissection proceeds inferiorly in a preseptal plane, separating the conjoined capsulopalpebral fascia and orbital septum. This plane is followed to the inferior orbital rim, where the periosteum is incised with preservation of a 3- to 4-mm cuff (**Fig. 1**). This marks the entry point to the subperiosteal plane. The conjunctival flap is draped over the cornea for protection.

If preoperative examination reveals excessive lid skin redundancy, a subciliary incision is utilized after canthotomy/cantholysis. The excision is extended laterally to join the crow's-feet incision. A suborbicularis plane is developed by dividing the muscle at an angle, preserving a cuff of pretarsal orbicularis. The skin-muscle flap is elevated to

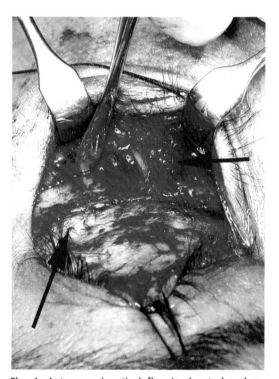

Fig. 1. A tarsoconjunctival flap is elevated and retracted superiorly to protect the cornea. The long arrow indicates the inferior orbital rim, whereas the short arrow points to condensations around the infraorbital nerve.

expose the middle lamella or orbital septum (**Fig. 2**). Dissection proceeds inferiorly to the inferior orbital rim, and the periosteum is incised (in the manner described previously) to access the subperiosteal plane.

The periosteum is elevated off the facial skeleton. Dissection boundaries are the gingivobuccal sulcus inferiorly, the malar eminence and medial insertion of the masseter laterally, and the nasomaxillary junction and pyriform aperture medially. Care should be taken to preserve the infraorbital (**Fig. 3**) and zygomaticofacial (**Fig. 4**) nerves as they exit their respective foramina. The infraorbital nerve should be completely skeletonized (see **Fig. 3**) and the orbital retaining ligament should be appropriately released and elevated to aid in mobilizing the midfacial tissues. An inferior periosteal incision is created near the gingivobuccal sulcus, and a clamp can be used to spread until superficial fat can be seen through the incision. This marks the full mobilization of the midface composite flap (**Fig. 5**), which, with superior traction, should be easily elevated without excessive force. To ensure proper mobility of the flap, lateral soft tissues should be swept away until the masseter origin is clearly visible.

A 3-0 Mersilene or polydioxanone suture is used to fixate the elevated soft tissues to the cuff of periosteum at the inferior orbital rim (**Fig. 6**). The sutures are placed through the inferior periosteum of the flap medial or lateral to the infraorbital nerve and pulled superiorly in the vector required to achieve the desired aesthetic effect (**Fig. 7**). The periosteum of the inferior orbital rim is frequently thicker and hardier at the inferolateral orbital rim, whereas the medial periorbita tends to not hold sutures as well. In patients with prominent tear trough deformities, a superomedial vector of elevation made be required. Bone-anchored

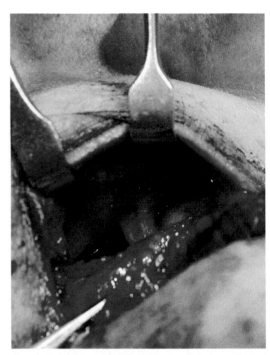

Fig. 3. Subperiosteal dissection medial, lateral, and inferior to the infraorbital nerve mobilizes soft tissue of the midface.

fixation devices, such as the Endotine Midface B implant (MicroAire, Charlottesville, Virginia) and the Mitek 2.0 mm TACIT anchor (DePuy Synthes, Warsaw, Indiana), are alternative fixation devices that can be used in this setting. The Endotine implant tines pierce the inferior periosteum and the implant tail is fixed superiorly to the bone below the inferior orbital rim using a resorbable screw. Suture fixation of soft tissues to the medial orbital rim can then be used to gently drape volume into the medial nasojugal trough.

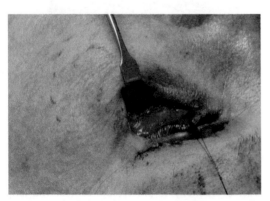

Fig. 2. A subciliary incision can be used to access the preseptal plane, which can be followed to the infraorbital rim.

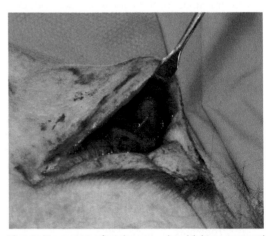

Fig. 4. Zygomaticofacial nerve should be preserved during dissection.

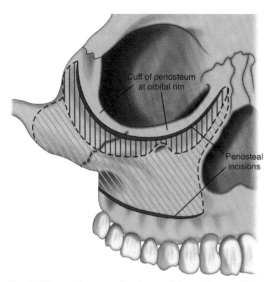

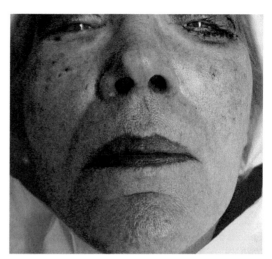

Fig. 7. Intraoperative view after elevation of left midface. The patient's left midface is seen at a higher level with a more aesthetic facial shape.

Fig. 5. The periosteum is elevated from the midface from the insertion of the masseter to the pyriform aperture. The tissues are mobilized from the periosteal incision at the orbital rim inferiorly to a periosteal incision at the gingivobuccal sulcus. (*From* Sclafani AP, Spalla TC. Surgical atlas of facial plastic surgery. New Delhi (India): Jaypee Brothers Medical Publishers (P) Ltd; 2014; with permission.)

The lateral canthus is then reconstructed using a 4-0 polytetrafluoroethylene suture from the lateral edge of the lateral canthal tendon to the internal aspect of the lateral orbital rim, at a position 2 to 3 mm superior to the original insertion. The canthotomy incision is closed with 6-0 fast absorbing gut suture. The edges of the transconjunctival incision should be realigned carefully. This incision does not require closure; however, if closure is performed, it should be done gently with 6-0 fast absorbing sutures without everting the wound edges. If skin resection is required, it should be done conservatively at this time using a pinch technique. If a skin muscle flap was used, the skin is redraped superiorly while the patient is asked to direct her vision in upgaze and open her mouth. Redundant skin is then carefully resected and the subciliary incision is closed with 6-0 chromic sutures. Postoperatively, no dressings are required, but cool compresses may be applied to the eyes and cheeks. These are applied intermittently for the first 24 to 36 hours. Eye lubricants are applied during the first postoperative week, and sutures are removed at 5 to 7 days.

DISCUSSION
Peripheral Versus Central Approaches

Early techniques for midface rejuvenation used peripheral-to-central dissections originating at traditional temporal and preauricular incisions. Centrofacial dissections subsequently developed from a desire to obtain a more natural-appearing lift. Elevation in a more vertical vector was theorized to more directly reverse the downward vectors of aging and additionally avoid the widened

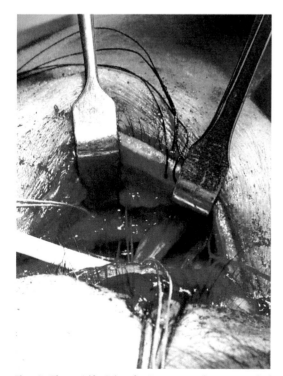

Fig. 6. The midfacial soft tissues can be suspended with Mersilene sutures to the periosteum at the orbital rim.

lateral sweep appearance that can occur with vectors that are too lateral. Central approaches also introduced a lower risk of facial nerve injury and disruption of vascular supply than peripheral dissections utilizing extensive dissection over the zygoma.[11] In the original description of the technique introduced by Hester and colleagues, direct vertical elevation and fixation of midfacial soft tissue was identified as a key principle of the subperiosteal cheek lift.[3,4] Multiple permutations of the original centrofacial approach now comprise the modern spectrum of midface lifting techniques.

Endoscopic Approaches

Endoscopic approaches to facelifting evolved from the pioneering studies of subperiosteal dissection and have since become important tools in facial rejuvenation. The use of endoscopes permits precise dissection and visualization of neurovascular structures, and the techniques are attractive to patients desiring minimally invasive procedures. The midface is often approached endoscopically in conjunction with the upper third of the face through temporal incisions, which is conceptually appealing because the forehead, brow, periocular region, and midface age together in a composite fashion. Ramirez[15] pioneered the extension of the endoscopic forehead lift to the midface, combining endoscopic dissection from the temporal region over the zygoma with midface access via blepharoplasty and Caldwell-Luc approaches. Dissection is carried out in a subperiosteal plane. Many surgeons have since established the safety and efficacy of these methods in rejuvenating the upper two-thirds of the face.[16–18] Benefits of endoscopic subperiosteal brow-midface lift can even be seen on the jawline and jowl regions in the lower third of the face.[18] The endoscopic malar pad lift utilizes a brow lift or crow's-foot incision to dissect in a suborbicularis plane just superficial to the zygomaticus major muscle to access and suspend the malar wad. Its primary benefit is improvement of the depth and contour of the nasolabial fold.[19] A transblepharoplasty endoscopic technique has been described in which an endoscope is passed through a lateral canthotomy incision and used to guide subperiosteal dissection and flap suspension using a vest-over-pants fixation technique. In this technique the vest of the superior periosteal cuff and superficial layer of deep temporal fascia is sutured over the superiorly elevated pants of the composite midface flap.[20] In the midface, endoscopic visualization may aid, in particular, the identification of the zygomaticofacial vessels and retaining ligaments, allowing precise release of relevant structures while avoiding injury to the facial nerve. A thorough understanding of facial anatomy is crucial to safely and effectively executing endoscopic approaches to the midface.

Planes of Dissection

Elevation of the midface can be performed in subcutaneous, suborbicularis or zygorbicular, or subperiosteal planes.[21] Subcutaneous plane dissection may not address the deeper structures contributing to the aged appearance and may lead to an excessively tightened appearance or reveal slight contour irregularities. Suborbicularis dissection can address a ptotic orbicularis muscle and malar fat pad and may best address difficult areas of the tear trough and nasolabial folds.[9,22] During dissection of the suborbicularis plane, is important to keep fat up off the periosteum during dissection in this plane to protect the branches of the facial nerve and zygomaticofacial nerves running within the SOOF to enter the periphery of the orbicularis muscle.[1,8] A 4- to 5-mm pretarsal cuff of orbicularis is also preserved to prevent microdenervation and orbicularis hypotonicity.[23] Techniques using both transconjunctival and subciliary incisions have been described to access this plane.[8,9,22] The zygorbicular plane extends this suborbicularis plane deep to the zygomaticus musculature. These may be more difficult planes of dissection, and some surgeons recommend transitioning to a subperiosteal plane if dissection within this plane cannot be maintained to protect the facial nerve.[8] The primary benefit of dissection of this plane is avoidance of the prolonged postoperative edema and chemosis that is known to accompany subperiosteal dissection (**Fig. 8**).

The described procedure demonstrates a dissection performed in the subperiosteal plane. Subperiosteal dissection is generally safe but leads to increased and prolonged postoperative edema and does not address rejuvenation of the neck when comprehensive rhytidectomy is planned. It provides excellent visualization of the infraorbital and zygomaticofacial nerves, aids in the protection of these structures as well as the facial nerve, and does not disrupt facial mimetic musculature. The periosteum is rich in lymphatic drainage, and disruption is theorized to cause the well-known prolonged facial edema and chemosis postoperatively, which has been reported to last up to 3 to 6 weeks. The authors' protocol is to administer intravenous dexamethasone prior to and near the end of the procedure, followed by a course of postoperative steroids. In the authors' experience, facial edema is rarely a significant patient concern after the first postoperative

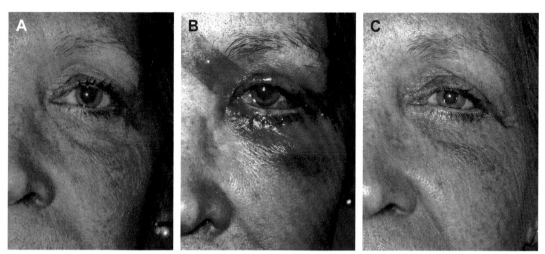

Fig. 8. Chemosis may delay healing and can lead to lid malposition unless adequate lid support is provided with canthoplasty or cnthopexy. (*A*) Preoperative, (*B*) 5-day postoperative, and (*C*) 8-week postoperative views.

week.[13,14] Elevating a composite flap with periosteal base allows for strong periosteum to bone or fascia fixation, typically to either the inferolateral orbital rim periosteum or the deep temporal fascia. This manipulation does not alter the relationship between the layered tissues of the composite flap. This is the reason some surgeons argue that subperiosteal elevation is ineffective at effacing the nasolabial fold, because it does not change the relative positions of the structures contributing to the fold.[9,10] This is commonly addressed using fillers or autogenous grafting material. Dissection of multiple planes may increase the amount of postoperative ecchymosis and edema as multiple layers of lymphatics and vasculature are traversed. The appropriate plane of dissection is heavily dependent on individual surgeon skill and experience. Dissection should be limited to the minimal amount necessary to address the severity of the midfacial ptosis.[4,21] Centrofacial rejuvenation approaches, therefore, can be applied to varying degrees of midface aging in a graduated and patient-specific manner, from simple extended blepharoplasty to partial or full midface elevation.[4]

The Tear Trough Deformity and the Suborbicularis Oculi Fat Lift Blepharoplasty

The tear trough deformity becomes apparent as soft tissues descend from the medial nasojugal area and can be difficult to address surgically. Fillers and autografts to this region are frequently used as adjuncts but may be limited in efficacy. Careful anatomic study by Freeman[9] suggested that inferior migration of the SOOF specifically contributes to the development of the tear trough. Its normal position is at the medial infraorbital rim

over the arcus marginalis, wrapped around the levator anguli oris muscle near its bony origin, and its descent skeletonizes this area, resulting in the tear trough. This anatomic finding is the basis for the SOOF lift blepharoplasty. This technique uses a transconjunctival approach with elevation and suspension of the SOOF to the arcus marginalis. Dissection is performed in a preperiosteal plane, and minimal excision of lower lid fat from the lateral fat compartment is performed. Freeman's initial study of 64 patients reported reliably good to excellent long-term results with specific regard to the nasojugal trough, and Freeman has since reported that this technique has become standard in his practice.[10,19] The superficial subciliary cheek described by Moelleken[22] is a similar procedure in that it achieves effective effacement of the tear trough using a suborbicularis plane of dissection. Arcus marginalis release can also be performed in the setting of an especially deep nasojugal fold. The use of dissection in a preperiosteal plane, as opposed to the subperiosteal plane, affords surgeons the ability to specifically alter the relative positions of the layered soft tissue structures of the midface. As discussed previously in regard to the nasolabial fold, this may underlie the failure of other techniques to adequately address the nasojugal deformity, particularly in subperiosteal approaches.

Management of the Lateral Canthus

Lower lid malpositions, such as lid retraction, scleral show, frank ectropion, and lateral canthal dystopia, represent a spectrum of postoperative sequelae that are among the most feared complications of transblepharoplasty techniques. Furthermore, surgical correction of lid malposition can be difficult. Focused preoperative evaluation can identify those patients at high risk for this outcome, such as patients with prominent globe/negative vector or patients with a history of prior blepharoplasty. The operative plan should anticipate lid retraction appropriately. Techniques, such as supraplacement of the canthoplasty and limiting the extent of dissection to prevent excessive edema, should be considered in these instances. It is paramount to avoid over-resection of skin and muscle of the lower lid, especially because superficial tissues bunch up with elevation of the midface. Some degree of apparent excess skin observed intraoperatively likely recovers its lost tone in the postoperative period, and pinch excisions may be performed at that time. A patient and conservative approach is thus warranted. In severe cases, spacer grafts from hard palate mucosa or ear cartilage also may be required to augment the posterior lamella if there is a deficiency of lid length either primarily or during a revision surgery. The technique chosen may also influence the risk of lid malposition—some surgeons have observed that a subperiosteal dissection may be associated with a higher incidence of ectropion.[23] Transconjunctival approaches theoretically offer advantages of less manipulation and scarring of the middle lamella[24,25] and reduced retracting forces on the eyelid due to division of the lower lid retractors of the posterior lamella. Additionally, a Frost suture may help counteract the downward traction of postoperative edema.

Hester and colleagues' original centrofacial transblepharoplasty procedure included a formal canthoplasty to prevent malposition based on previous work in lower eyelid blepharoplasty, but complications directly related to canthoplasty, such as canthal webbing or notching requiring revision, were observed.[3,4,6] Patipa[24,25] observed that a vast majority of patients with midface descent exhibit lateral canthal tendon laxity and, therefore, require canthotomy/cantholysis and tendon reattachment. In all instances of canthotomy and/or cantholysis, careful reconstruction of the lateral commissure is essential to achieving a good outcome.

Other investigators think that although canthus and lid support are essential, a formal canthotomy is not routinely necessary because it disrupts the smooth shape of the lower eyelid and may lead to complications of its own. In 1999, Gunter and Hackney modified the procedure described by Hester and colleagues to avoid including routine lateral canthoplasty in appropriate patients and reported excellent results on 62 patients, with a similar rate of lower lid complications.[6] Some investigators argue along similar lines that patients with normal lid position and tension preoperatively do not require any additional lid support, because midface elevation alone provides adequate support for the lower lid.[12] A 10-year review of lower blepharoplasties with lateral canthal support supported routine use of canthal support in the form of canthoplasty, canthopexy, or orbicularis arc suspension, and this work has been corroborated throughout the literature by the experiences of other surgeons.[26] Canthopexy and other more conservative techniques have proved effective at stabilizing the lateral canthus while avoiding a formal canthotomy/cantholysis in appropriately selected patients with mild lid laxity.[6,8,10,26,27] Experience has shown that postoperative lower lid position may be more dependent on cheek elevation and fixation and appropriate skin excision than on surgical alteration of the lateral canthus, and a trend favoring canthopexy without canthotomy in appropriate patients has evolved.[4] Ultimately, surgeon skill and experience may be the most relevant factors in managing the lower lid and lateral canthus.

Restoring Facial Volume

Facial volume loss and bony remodeling are gaining increasing appreciation as major contributors to the stigmata of facial aging. Augmentation techniques, such as cheek or submalar implants, can be considered for restoring these deficits, with thoughtful placement to avoid increased intermalar distance or the praying mantis deformity. These options may be more appropriate particularly for patients who congenitally lack midfacial soft tissue or have bony hypoplasia or patients with severe facial wasting, because midface lifting procedures simply redistribute soft tissue volume to areas of relative deficit. Midface lifting may be contraindicated in these patients for whom implants or other augmentation procedures are more appropriate.[14,28] A review of surgical outcomes of 150 midface rejuvenation patients by Jacono and Ransom[28] showed that a hypoplastic facial skeleton and loss of skin elasticity were the most important statistically significant predictors of poor outcome as measured by patient dissatisfaction. Pigmentation changes or static rhytids may benefit from concomitant laser resurfacing or chemical peels, with conservative pinch technique skin and muscle excision reserved for skin irregularities proved refractory to these treatments. Excessive skin laxity may require full rhytidectomy.

Additional local volumizing techniques may be used to fine-tune a midface lifting procedure. Fillers, autologous free fat or SMAS grafts, or allografts can be transferred to the tear trough area or

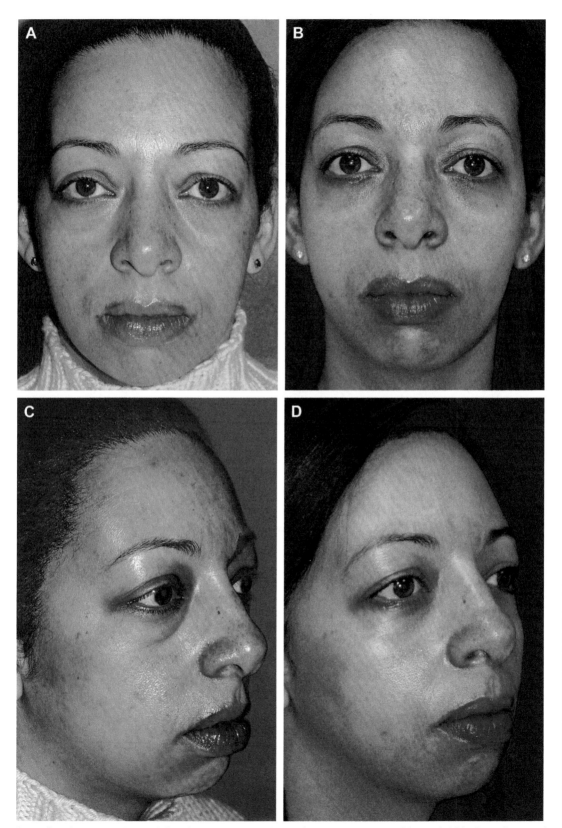

Fig. 9. (A, C) Preoperative and (B, D) postoperative views after transconjunctival lower lid blepharoplasty and transpalpebral midface lift.

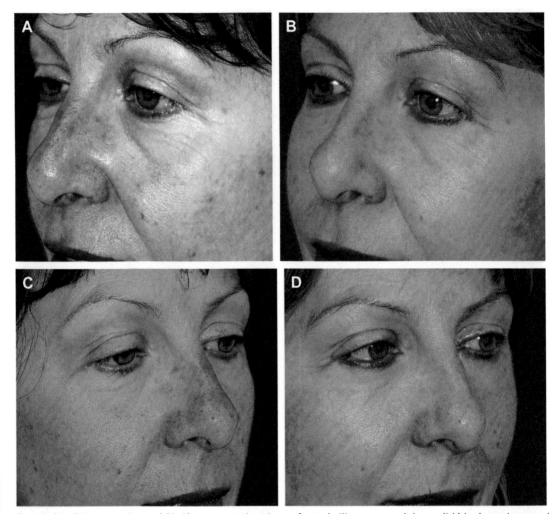

Fig. 10. (*A, C*) Preoperative and (*B, D*) postoperative views after subciliary approach lower lid blepharoplasty and transpalpebral midface lift.

nasolabial folds, which can be difficult to fully correct surgically. Care should be taken to avoid areas of thin skin flaps during these procedures, because grafting in these areas may result in noticeable surface irregularities.

HARMONIOUS REJUVENATION

Centrofacial transpalpebral approaches to the midface offer patients and surgeons the ability to achieve a more natural rejuvenation that can be performed in isolation in appropriately selected patients or as part of an overall rejuvenation plan. These techniques offer a unique approach to the tear trough and malar mound deformities of the midface and address the lower eyelid and cheek as a unit (**Figs. 9** and **10**). When used in conjunction with appropriately selected fillers, implants, and autologous grafts, these techniques can

address the more difficult area of the nasolabial fold or can be used in cases of severe facial volume deficiency. Comprehensive preoperative evaluation should also include assessment of the brows, jawline, and neck, because the midface does not age on its own. In particular, the brow, upper eyelid, and lower eyelid/midface age together in a composite manner. It is important, therefore, to keep in mind that transpalpebral midface lift techniques do not replace rhytidectomy and that a multifaceted and patient-specific approach to facial rejuvenation should be the surgical mandate.

SUPPLEMENTARY DATA

Supplementary data related to this article can be found online at http://dx.doi.org/10.1016/j.fsc.2015.01.007.

REFERENCES

1. Mendelson BC, Muzaffar AR, Adams WP Jr. Surgical anatomy of the midcheek and malar mounds. Plast Reconstr Surg 2002;110(3):885–96.

2. Muzaffar AR, Mendleson BC, Adams WP Jr. Surgical anatomy of the ligamentous attachments of the lower lid and lateral canthus. Plast Reconstr Surg 2002;110(3):885–96.

3. Hester TR, Codner MA, McCord CD. The "centrofacial" approach for correction of facial aging using the transblepharoplasty subperiosteal cheek lift. Aesthet Surg J 1996;16:51–8.

4. Hester TR Jr, Codner MA, McCord CD, et al. Evolution of technique of the direct transblepharoplasty approach for the correction of lower lid and midfacial aging: maximizing results and minimizing complications in a 5-year experience. Plast Reconstr Surg 2000;105:393–406.

5. Paul MD, Calvert JW, Evans GR. The evolution of the midface lift in aesthetic plastic surgery. Plast Reconstr Surg 2006;117:1809–27.

6. Gunter JP, Hackney FL. A simplified transblepharoplasty subperiosteal cheek lift. Plast Reconstr Surg 1999;103:2029–35.

7. Cintra H. Is the transpalpebral approach to the upper and midface rejuvenation a safe method?. In: de Castro CC, Boehm K, Codner MA, editors. Techniques in aesthetic plastic surgery series: midface surgery. Saunders Elsevier Ltd; 2009. p. 133–47.

8. Few JW, Llorente O. Transconjunctival deep-plane midface rejuvenation. In: de Castro CC, Boehm K, Codner MA, editors. Techniques in aesthetic plastic surgery series: midface surgery. Saunders Elsevier Ltd; 2009. p. 161–71.

9. Freeman MS. Transconjunctival sub-orbicularis oculi fat (soof) pad lift blepharoplasty: a new technique for the effacement of nasojugal deformity. Arch Facial Plast Surg 2000;2:16–21.

10. Freeman MS. Rejuvenation of the midface. Facial Plast Surg 2003;19(2):223–36.

11. Boehm KA, Codner MA. Evolution of the superiosteal midface lift. In: de Castro CC, Boehm K, Codner MA, editors. Techniques in aesthetic plastic surgery series: midface surgery. Saunders Elsevier Ltd; 2009. p. 105–18.

12. LaFerriere KA, Kilpatrick JK. Transblepharoblasty: subperiosteal approach to rejuvenation of the aging midface. Facial Plast Surg 2003;19(2):157–70.

13. Sclafani AP. Midface lift. In: Sclafani AP, Spalla T, editors. Surgical techniques in otolaryngology-head & neck surgery: facial plastic & reconstructive surgery. 1st edition. New Delhi (India: Jaypee Brothers Medical Publishers (P) Ltd; 2014. p. 65–72.

14. Sclafani AP. The Multivectorial subperiosteal midface lift. Facial Plast Surg 2001;17(1):29–36.

15. Ramirez OM. Endoscopic full facelift. Aesthetic Plast Surg 1994;18:363–71.

16. Quatela VC, Azzi JP, Antunes M. Endoscopic-assisted facelifting. Facial Plast Surg 2014;30:413–21.

17. DeFatta RJ, Williams EF III. Midface lifting: current standards. Facial Plast Surg 2011;27:77–85.

18. Batniji RK, Williams EF III. Effects of subperiosteal midfacial elevation via an endoscopic brow-lift incision on lower facial rejuvenation. Facial Plast Surg 2005;21:33–7.

19. Freeman MS. Endoscopic techniques for rejuvenation of the midface. Facial Plast Surg Clin North Am 2005;13:141–55.

20. Williams JV. Transblepharoplasty endoscopic subperiosteal midface lift. Plast Reconstr Surg 2002;110(7):1769–75.

21. Keller GK, Quatela VC, Antunes MB, et al. Midface lift: panel discussion. Facial Plast Surg Clin North Am 2014;22:119–37.

22. Moelleken BR. The superficial subciliary cheek lift, a technique for rejuvenating the infraorbital region and nasojugal groove: a clinical series of 71 patients. Plast Reconstr Surg 1999;104:1863–74.

23. Moelleken BR. Midfacial rejuvenation. Facial Plast Surg 2003;19(2):209–21.

24. Papita M. Transblepharoplasty lower eyelid and midface rejuvenation: part I. Avoiding complications by utilizing lessons learned from the treatment of complications. Plast Reconstr Surg 2004;113:1459–68.

25. Patipa M. Transblepharoplasty lower eyelid and midface rejuvenation: part II. Functional applications of midface elevation. Plast Reconstr Surg 2004;113:1469–74.

26. Codner MA, Wolfli JN, Anzarut A. Primary transcutaneous lower blepharoplasty with routine lateral canthal support: a comprehensive 10-year review. Plast Reconstr Surg 2008;121:241–50.

27. Faigen S. Algorithm for canthoplasty: the lateral retinacular suspension: a simplified suture canthopexy. Plast Reconstr Surg 1999;103(7):2042–53.

28. Jacono AA, Ransom ER. Anatomic predictors of unsatisfactory outcomes in surgical rejuvenation of the midface. JAMA Facial Plast Surg 2013;15(2):101–9.

Midface Sculpting with Autologous Fat

Lesley A. Rabach, MD[a],*, Robert A. Glasgold, MD[b,c], Samuel M. Lam, MD[d],
Mark J. Glasgold, MD[b,c]

KEYWORDS

- Fat grafting • Aging face • Volume loss • Midface

KEY POINTS

- There is currently a major paradigm shift from purely excision-based surgery to combined surgical and volume enhancement.
- Because there is still no perfect facial filler, development of synthetic facial injectables continue to advance at a remarkable pace.
- Each type of filler carries a specific characteristic that makes it more suitable for a certain clinical application.
- The continuing change in facial fillers offers the possibility for volume augmentation procedures with less downtime and without the need for harvesting fat.
- We predict that volume enhancement will continue to play an increasing role as both a complementary procedure and as a stand-alone procedure in facial rejuvenation.

INTRODUCTION

Over the past several years, the role of volume restoration with autologous fat has become an increasingly recognized entity as a primary mechanism by which to overcome the aging process. Facial fat grafting has assumed a renewed interest among aesthetic surgeons owing to technical advances that have been shown to be beneficial both in achieving consistently excellent cosmetic results and in limiting morbidity.[1]

The aging process can be understood with a simple analogy of the aging face: in youth, the face is like a grape, and as people age, volume depletion causes the face to become like a raisin. When performing age-related surgeries, the redundant skin is lifted, pulled, and cut away so that the remainder no longer resembles the grape of youth but is more like a truncated pea.

This approach does not restore all the highlights, contours, and convexities of youth. Filling the depressed facial zones helps restore a youthful appearance more effectively. Note that this reductionist philosophy does not reflect the authors' opinion entirely, because we recognize the complexity of the aging process that can comprise volume loss, volume gain, gravitational descent, and dermatologic changes. In the past, the aging face was perceived as a change caused by gravity and skin redundancy and it is now interpreted as arising from tissue deflation, which can be corrected with facial fat grafting.[2]

The best approach for prospective patients with aging faces seeking to restore a youthful countenance is to view old photographs from the patient's youth. Old photographs provide a framework for our goals and help the patient understand what combination of procedures will provide a

Disclosures: The authors have no disclosures.
[a] Private Practice, 224 Riverside Drive #3D, New York, NY 10025, USA; [b] Robert Wood Johnson Medical School, Rutgers University, New Brunswick, NJ, USA; [c] Private Practice, 31 River Road, Highland, Park, NJ 08904, USA; [d] Willow Bend Wellness Center, 6101 Chapel Hill Boulevard, Suite 101, Plano, TX 75093, USA
* Corresponding author.
E-mail address: lesleyrabach@gmail.com

natural and rejuvenated appearance. During the consultation and evaluation, it is important to maintain a global approach for optimal rejuvenation. The myriad of procedures may include fat grafting, face-lifting, microliposuction/liposuction, blepharoplasty, and or skin therapies. The combination approach toward fat grafting is not necessarily a stand-alone procedure in every case but an adjuvant to traditional procedures (**Fig. 1**).[3] This integrated strategy allows the surgeon to select the right combination of individually tailored procedures based on how that person looked previously.

The advent of disposable microcannulas for use with office-based facial fillers, and the continued development of filler products intended for facial volumization, has challenged fat grafting as the sole method for facial volumization. Fillers are now a suitable alternative in patients who desire fat transfer or as an adjunct to fat transfer because microcannulas can be used for advanced facial sculpting, which fat grafting alone was only able to achieve a few years ago.[3]

This article proposes a systematic approach to facial fat enhancement of the midface emphasizing simplicity, consistency, and safety, which is the result of a decade of clinical experience with ongoing refinements in technique. Autologous fat transfer plays a critical role in facial rejuvenation of the midface as a stand-alone

procedure or in combination with traditional age-related surgeries.[4] Preoperative education and counseling are emphasized.

TREATMENT GOALS AND PLANNED OUTCOMES

There are several goals of facial fat grafting. These goals include the achievement of a natural rejuvenation and restoration of youth, the avoidance of complications, and the attainment of long-lasting aesthetic benefit. In the modern era of facial fat grafting, learning about autologous fat grafting requires completely rethinking of the approach to the aging face. Clinicians must use a novel aesthetic appreciation of the aging process. Clinicians also must use new operative techniques, including body harvesting and infiltration, and must manage unique complications.[5] The details of approach and technique are described later.

Facial aesthetic surgeons must think about autologous fat transfer in a different manner than a typical operative procedure. Specifically, typically they strive for the ideal result; however, for autologous fat transfer, a more conservative approach is advocated.[6] Surgeons must taper their expectations. In particular, as the limit of fat transfer is pushed by increasing volumes transferred to obtain an ideal result, the associated increased recovery time and potential for

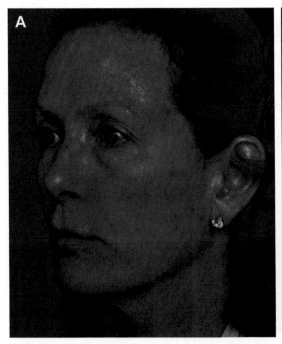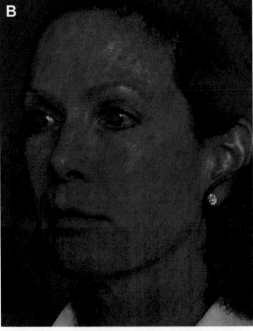

Fig. 1. (*A*, *B*) Combination approach to fat grafting. Upper and lower eyelid blepharoplasty was performed with fat transfer to the upper eyelid, lower eyelid, cheek, submalar and buccal regions. (*Photo courtesy* of Robert Glasgold, MD. *Reprinted* with permission from Glasgold Group Plastic Surgery, 2012.)

complications increase dramatically. If the surgeon or patient thinks that they is undercorrected, reharvest and transfer of additional fat is an easy task compared with the difficulty of correcting a complication such as a visible contour irregularity or reduction of an overcorrected face. Thus, conservatism should be the rule, especially for surgeons inexperienced with facial fat grafting.

The aesthetic of volume enhancement embodied by facial fat grafting mandates a different approach to patients. The goal of facial fat transfer is to return patients back to their own youthful appearances. Many aesthetic surgeons now evaluate a patient during consultation and attempt to define what areas of the face require improvement without reference to how the patient looked when younger. Patients are encouraged to bring in young photographs, which help the surgeon evaluate the patient's youthful appearance and help the patient understand the importance of volume loss in the aging process and the need to replace it. The patient must help guide the desired aesthetic outcome. Regardless, patients' past photographs are reviewed to help the patients understand the role of fat grafting. Past photographs also help surgeons to conceptualize the optimal fat grafting plan.

Our vision for facial rejuvenation does not insist that autologous fat transfer is the only possible method by which facial enhancement is achieved. Fat grafting is a complementary role in our clinical practice. We think that a patient's aesthetic result can be greatly enhanced by the use of a combination of approaches; for example, fat grafting, face-lifting, and blepharoplasty (**Fig. 2**). Patients are considerably more pleased when each procedure adds to the tally of aesthetic improvement. Traditional procedures and fat transfer need not be exclusive of one another. Two ideologies can be embraced: volume enhancement for volume depletion and lifting procedures for gravitational descent. Judicious use of fat grafting with select lifting procedures can constitute a potent mixture for correcting specific flaws of aging. Combining procedures can also diminish the risk of morbidity. With ongoing clinical experience, surgeons will begin to perceive the role that volume enhancement can play in the armamentarium of facial rejuvenation.

ANATOMY

As the face matures, soft tissue loss is accentuated by the presence of facial retaining ligaments

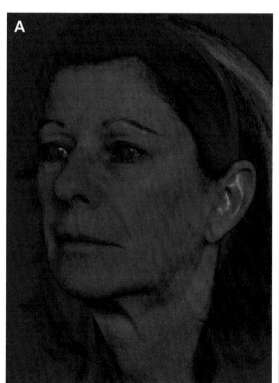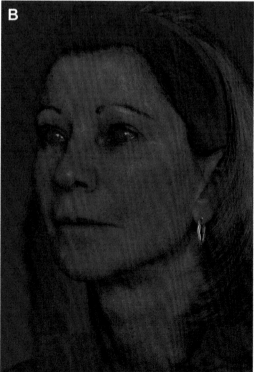

Fig. 2. (*A, B*) Fat grafting to the upper eyelid, lower eyelid, and cheek, performed in combination with face-lift, and upper and lower eyelid blepharoplasty. (*Photo courtesy* of Robert Glasgold, MD. *Reprinted* with permission from Glasgold Group Plastic Surgery, 2012.)

that create unfavorable shadows. The anatomy for fat grafting does not relate so much to an intimate knowledge of specific underlying anatomic structures but rather to understanding the hills and valleys across the surface of the face that can be transformed into a more uniformly convexity free of unwanted depressions.[7]

The easiest way to categorize the face for anatomic understanding is into thirds: the upper third comprises the brow and temple area; the middle third comprises the cheek and midface; and the lower third comprises the prejowl, jowl, and lateral mandible. This systematic approach provides a formula for specific volume enhancement based on each individual anatomic territory. Rather than delve into the esoteric minutiae related to each anatomic zone, the clinical significance of each area is emphasized with attention to the clinically relevant pearls to guide the optimal surgical strategy.

The middle third of the face is perhaps the most important area for facial rejuvenation with autologous fat and is anatomically the most complex in terms of fully understanding each subunit. By our definition, the middle facial third includes the lower eyelid, malar, and submalar area. A youthful face is characterized by a confluence of the lower eyelid and cheek regions, which become separated into visually distinct regions with the aging process. With aging, the orbital rim becomes a separate entity from the cheek because of orbital fat bulging superiorly and the cheek fat receding, which reveals the bony orbital rim.[3,8] The voluminous lateral cheek mound of youth dissipates to uncover a smaller, flatter contour of the malar bony eminence that lacks any notable soft tissue coverage. The anterior cheek begins to separate, often with a linear depression that courses from the nasojugal depression down inferolaterally to the buccal recess, which corresponds with the ligamentous attachment known as the malar septum (**Fig. 3**).[9] The buccal region can show marked atrophy and should be reconstituted along with the discussed anterior and lateral malar regions to achieve better confluence and to avoid exaggeration of buccal hollowing following malar augmentation. As an extension of the midface, the nasolabial fold should be deemed part of midfacial volume enhancement.

PREOPERATIVE PLANNING AND PREPARATION

The facial fat transfer consultation is different than the discussion of lifting style procedures. In order to have a rewarding consultation, the surgeon and patient must be in concordance. Thus, it is imperative to encourage review of older

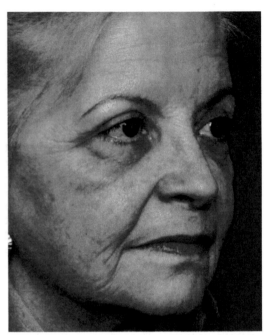

Fig. 3. The anterior cheek separating with a linear depression. (*From* Lam SM, Glasgold MJ, Glasgold RA. Complementary fat grafting. Philadelphia: Lippincott Williams & Wilkins, 2007; with permission.)

photographs as an instrument to discuss restoration of youth because a patient may not initially entirely understand the benefits of autologous fat. Reviewing each decade of change and showing the gradual dissipation of soft tissue volume as seen in prior photographs, a patient can begin to truly appreciate the aesthetic objectives.[7] In addition, showing before-and-after photographs of other patients who have similar anatomy and who have benefited from autologous facial fat transfer can also be illuminating to a prospective patient. In addition, after establishing realistic aesthetic objectives, the surgeon must ensure that the patient fully comprehends the benefits and limitations of the procedure.

PROCEDURAL APPROACH
Marking the Recipient Sites

The patient should be in an upright position so that all the folds and depressions can be easily visualized. Rather than a standard gentian violet marking pen, a permanent marker is advocated owing to the ease of removing the marks shortly after the procedure is completed. The planned areas to be augmented with fat are outlined. Often this includes the temple, superior and inferior orbital rim, anterior and lateral cheek, buccal hollow, precanine fossa, nasolabial groove, prejowl sulcus, and anterior chin (**Fig. 4**).

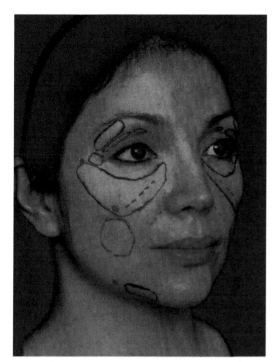

Fig. 4. The planned areas to be augmented with fat are outlined. (*From* Lam SM, Glasgold MJ, Glasgold RA. Complementary fat grafting. Philadelphia: Lippincott Williams & Wilkins, 2007; with permission.)

Selection of Donor Site

Donor-site selection is based on where there is available fat for harvesting and on fat viability.[10] It also depends on the level of anesthesia and the ease of harvesting relative to patient positioning. Asking the individual where the most abundant adipose reserves are located is the easiest method for selecting the favored donor site for fat harvesting. Although men typically carry their extra fat in the truncal distribution, women's fat storage can be either truncal or extremity dominant. The lower abdomen serves as a good source in both men and women and is a site easily accessed without patient repositioning. When evaluating the lower abdomen as a potential donor site, patients should be examined to rule out the presence of abdominal hernias. In women the outer thigh often provides an excellent and abundant source of fat; alternatively the inner thigh can be used, which offers the benefit of not requiring intraoperative repositioning. In men, the hip is a good alternative for fat harvest but requires intraoperative patient repositioning.

Anesthesia and General Considerations

Fat grafting can be undertaken with almost any level of anesthesia, from straight local anesthesia to general anesthesia. Intravenous conscious sedation is our preferred anesthesia, because it provides the best balance of patient comfort and sedation, and facilitates intraoperative patient repositioning as necessary. In instances of small-volume secondary fat transfers, the procedure is generally performed with an oral benzodiazepine and local anesthetic. The patient's donor and recipient sites are prepared in a sterile fashion using povidone-iodine solution and sterile drapes. If other concurrent procedures are being performed, facial fat transfer should be performed first because, theoretically, the longer the tissue is outside the patient, the less viable the fat graft becomes.

Donor-site Harvesting

The donor site is anesthetized once the patient achieves an appropriate level of sedation. An injection of 20 mL of 0.25% lidocaine with 1:400,000 epinephrine is infiltrated with a 17.8-mm (7-inch) 22-gauge spinal needle placing half in the superficial aspect of the fat pad (the immediate subcutaneous plane) and the other half in the deep aspect of the fat pad (above the fascia in the deep subcutaneous plane). The 20-mL mixture of anesthetic solution can be constituted by mixing 15 mL of normal saline with 5 mL of 1% lidocaine with 1:100,000 epinephrine. For individuals who are under lighter sedation or straight local anesthesia, a 50:50 mix of 10 mL of normal saline and 10 mL of 1% lidocaine with 1:100,000 epinephrine is used instead. A total of 20 mL of anesthetic mixture can be used for the entire lower abdomen, whereas 20 mL per extremity donor site is preferred.

After an appropriate time for anesthesia has elapsed, a 16-gauge Nokor™ needle is used to create a stab incision through which the harvesting cannula can be inserted. Fat harvesting is undertaken with a blunt bullet-tip cannula (Tulip Medical Inc, San Diego, CA) attached to a Luer-Lok™ 10-mL syringe. Harvesting is performed with hand suction, retracting the plunger with approximately 2 mL of negative pressure to minimize trauma to the adipocytes: a retaining device, such as a Johnnie Lok™ (Tulip Medical Inc) is useful for maintaining negative pressure and reduces unnecessary forearm strain. As the cannula traverses the fat pad, dimpling of the overlying skin, which indicates being too superficial, should not be seen. Harvesting should be focused on getting fat from the mid to deeper levels of the fat pad. The nondominant hand can be used to stabilize the fat pad but should not pinch or tent the skin, which can lead to uneven fat harvesting. In general, surgeons should ensure that the same area of the fat pad is not being over harvested. After the cannula is passed back and forth in a prescribed area, the cannula should be retracted back almost to the entry site before redirecting the cannula into a fresh adjacent site. This maneuver ensures that the cannula does not remain in the same harvesting site, thereby allowing uniform harvesting across the donor site and preventing iatrogenic contour irregularities. Estimation of the amount of fat needed for harvest should be based on the assumption that about half of the collected volume will be fat, with the remainder consisting of blood, lysed fat cells, and lidocaine, which will be separated out during fat purification.

Fat Processing

After the fat has been harvested into the 10-mL Luer-Lok™ syringes, the fat is prepared by centrifugation or by Puregraft® (Puregraft, San Diego, Ca). Fat processing is performed on a sterile field. Although the centrifuge is off the sterile field, sterile sleeves, within which the 10-mL syringes sit, are used to maintain sterility. A dedicated plug and cap (Tulip Medical Inc) must be attached to each syringe to avoid spillage of contents during the centrifugation process. Many centrifuge models exist that can accommodate sterile sleeves or insertable rotary trays to maintain the sterility of the syringes. The syringes are inserted into the centrifuge in a balanced distribution and spun at approximately 3000 revolutions per minute for 3 minutes. On removal, the supernatant (on the non–Luer-Lok™ side) containing the lysed fatty acids is poured off first into a gauze or waste basin. Only after the supranatant is poured off should the bloody infranatant be drained from the Luer-Lok™ side. Inadvertently draining the infranatant first predisposes the column of fat to slide out of the other side of the syringe when pouring off the supranatant. The syringe, which now contains only a column of purified fat, is placed into a test tube rack or cup so that it stands upright. A noncut 4 × 4 cotton gauze or neuropaddie is inserted into the syringe in contact with the fat in order to wick away the excess supranatant for a period of 5 to 10 minutes. The contents from several 10-mL syringes are then transferred to an empty 20-mL syringe from the open non-Luer-Lok_ to the open Luer-Lokside. The plunger is then inserted into the back of the 20-mL syringe.

Puregraft® is a membrane filtration system for processing fat developed by Cytori therapeutics as part of the technology for isolating adipose-derived stem cells. Puregraft® uses dual filtration to purify fat. After fat is removed using the process earlier, the Puregraft® system (50-mL or 250-mL bags) is set up and fat is injected into the fat port of the Puregraft® bag. Lactated Ringer solution is infiltrated into the bag (2 times the volume of fat), the Puregraft® bag is agitated for a specified amount of time, placed flat for 1 minute, and then the wash fluid is drained through the drain port. This process is performed 2 times until fat is purified of free lipids and other contaminants. Purified fat is then removed with a 20-mL Luer-Lok syringe through the tissue port for reinjection.

Regardless of the chosen processing technique, the fat is then transferred from the 20-mL Luer-Lok syringe, using a Luer-Lok hub, into individual 1-mL Luer-Lok syringes. Fat injections are performed using the 1-mL syringes attached to a 0.9-mm or 1.2-mm blunt spoon-tip cannula (Tulip Medical Inc).

Injection Techniques

In order to increase the likelihood of fat survival, only small parcels of fat (0.03–0.1 mL) are infiltrated per pass of the cannula across multiple tissue planes. The 3 tissue planes (referred to later) are deep, middle, and superficial, corresponding respectively with a supraperiosteal plane, a midfascial to deep subcutaneous plane, and a superficial subcutaneous plane. Although these are not distinct visualized planes, their importance is for guiding fat placement in such away that fat survival can be maximized and contour problems minimized.

The amount of fat injected per pass of the cannula varies from 0.03 to 0.1 mL depending on the area treated. There are generally 4 major sites of entry for the cannula, referred to earlier as entry sites A, B, C, and D. Additional entry sites should be used as needed to address the desired areas of augmentation. Entry site A is located at the mid-cheek approximately at the base of the malar septal depression. Entry site B resides about 2 cm lateral to the lateral canthus, C is situated immediately behind the prejowl sulcus at the anterior border of the jowl, and D is located just above the brow to address the superior orbital rim (Fig. 5). Each entry site is made with a standard 20-gauge needle through which the blunt infiltration cannula can be inserted.

Before fat infiltration, the entry and recipient sites need to be anesthetized with 1% lidocaine with 1:100,000 epinephrine. The entry sites and field blocks are done with a 30-gauge and 27-gauge needle respectively. The recipient sites are also infiltrated diffusely with the same anesthetic using a blunt infiltration cannula. Use of the same blunt infiltration cannula for fat infiltration for local anesthetic can minimize the likelihood of ecchymosis. In general, 5 to 10 mL of lidocaine are sufficient to achieve adequate anesthesia each side of the face.

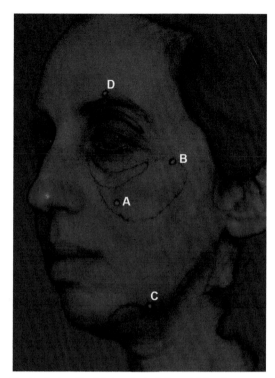

Fig. 5. Entry site A is located at the midcheek approximately at the base of the malar septal depression. Entry site B resides about 2 cm lateral to the lateral canthus, C is situated immediately behind the prejowl sulcus at the anterior border of the jowl, and D is located just above the brow to address the superior orbital rim. (*From* Glasgold RA, Glasgold MJ, Lam SA. In: Papel I, editor. Facial plastic and reconstructive surgery, 4th edition. New York: Thieme; in press.)

Volume loss in the midface results in visible breakpoints along the malar septum and between the lower lid and cheek, imparting an aged and tired appearance. Often, the midface is the most important region of the face to augment with fat. Reestablishing a uniform and seamless contour between the lower eyelid and cheek should be the principal objective in many cases. As previously mentioned, although infiltration of fat into the canine fossa and nasolabial fold is unlikely to efface a deep nasolabial fold, it is important for the purpose of creating a better transition between the newly augmented cheek and the upper lip.[9]

The inferior orbital rim is one of the most difficult areas of the face to enhance with fat and constitutes a region where the most complications arise. Injection of too large a fat bolus (>0.03–0.05 mL per cannula pass) or placement of fat too superficially increases the chance of a noticeable irregularity postoperatively. The most important change in technique, which has reduced complications dramatically, is an inferiorly based entry site so

the cannula passes perpendicularly to the inferior orbital rim. This maneuver should be performed with the index finger of the surgeon's nondominant hand placed on the superior aspect of the inferior orbital rim to protect the globe. As the surgeon begins incorporating fat transfer, it is recommended that a conservative amount of fat be placed along the inferior orbital rim (a total of 2 mL per side) in the immediately supraperiosteal plane so as to minimize contour problems. As surgeons gain experience with the technique they will find that larger volumes of fat can be used with additional placement in a more superficial plane to allow for optimal results, particularly in the most volume-deficient patients. The lateral and anterior cheeks are easy areas to augment with fat, allowing more superficial passage of the cannula with the more generous amount of 0.1 mL per pass without risking contour irregularities. The skeletonized lateral cheek should be augmented to restore a youthful, full, rounded contour that blends well with a full anterior cheek. The anterior cheek is typically divided by a linear depression running from the superomedial nasojugal groove to the inferolateral buccal region. Placement of fat into the anterior cheek should principally be situated into the greatest areas of tissue loss: the depression at the malar septum and the region inferomedial to the malar septum. Passage of the cannula to reach the anterior cheek can be made from a lateral cheek entry site, and the cannula often must be forcefully pushed through the fibrous malar septum to breach it. At times, the malar septum does not pose much resistance and can easily be traversed. Patients should be evaluated for the presence of a malar bag, which appears as a protuberance at the junction of the anterior and lateral cheek lying just lateral to the upper portion of the malar septum. When present, surgeons should attempt to avoid placement of excessive fat under the already prominent malar bag. Gentle contouring around the malar bag can help soften the appearance of the malar protuberance while at the same time rebuilding the lost volume of the cheek. If patients note a history of fluctuating, cyclical edema of the malar bag, placement of fat immediately below this structure may only worsen the condition and lead to a protracted swelling in this area for several months. In thin patients, the buccal and submalar regions are often hollow and can tolerate a generous amount of fat with minimal concern of contour irregularity. Placement of fat into the subcutaneous tissue and more deeply softens a gaunt appearance and provides a better transition between the malar and submalar regions. In addition, the canine fossa and the nasolabial fold are augmented with fat, not with the expectation of effacement of the fold but again to achieve an improved transition between the newly augmented anterior cheek and the upper lip. A generous amount of fat can be placed into the canine fossa (the triangular depression circumscribed by the nasal ala medially and the upper extent of the nasolabial fold laterally) deeply into the supraperiosteal plane to improve the hollowness in this area. The entire nasolabial fold, including the canine fossa, can then be augmented from a perpendicular direction into a more superficial subcutaneous plane.

POTENTIAL COMPLICATIONS AND MANAGEMENT

The complications that arise after fat grafting are more distinctive than those that arise after traditional lifting procedures. Injuries to nerves or vascular structures are extremely rare and are beyond the scope of this article. A classification of complications following fat grafting, including lumps, bulges, overcorrection, under-correction, and entry-site divot, is presented here.

Lumps

Lumps are small, discrete areas of excessive fat, and are most likely to occur in the periorbital region because of the thin soft tissue covering in the region. Technically it is caused by either too large a bolus of fat with a single pass or too much fat placed in one spot, instead of appropriately dispersing the small parcels throughout the region. Conservative placement of fat in the periorbital regions is an important step in avoiding this problem. When a lump does occur, treatment begins with steroid injections into the area of concern. If this fails to correct the problem, and there appears to be a discrete lump of fat, directly excising this can alleviate the contour deformity. If this proves ineffective the definitive remedy is excision of the lump through a discrete incision situated along the inferior orbital rim at the junction of the thin lower lid skin and the thicker cheek skin (**Fig. 6**).

Bulges

A bulge is a wide contour irregularity, characterized by palpable persistent edema or thickening. A bulge generally manifests as an oval-shaped elevation with palpable induration oriented parallel to the inferior orbital rim.

Injection with conservative amounts of triamcinolone acetonide in increasing strengths from 5 mg/mL to 40 mg/mL repeated over 1 to 2 months have been shown to be beneficial in most circumstances. In our experience, direct liposuction of these areas has not been successful.

Overcorrection

Overcorrection is a difficult condition to correct and should be avoided at all cost. As previously discussed, a conservative strategy for autologous fat transfer should be instituted to prevent this problem from arising. It is common in the early postoperative period for patients to be concerned that too much fat was placed. Patients are informed of significant tissue edema and thus time must pass for resorption of nonviable adipocytes before results can truly be appreciated. For this reason we recommend waiting 6 months before considering any surgical intervention to address overcorrection. Correction of this entity involves microliposuction of the areas perceived to be overcorrected using an 18-gauge Klein-Capistrano microliposuction cannula in a cross-hatched pattern.

Undercorrection

Undercorrection is the best complication to encounter, because it is the most easily correctable condition. Because of the variable survival of transferred adipocytes, we counsel all patients preoperatively of the possible need for a touch-up procedure to achieve the desired end point. Additional fat harvesting and infiltration can be accomplished quickly and without difficulty under local anesthesia or limited intravenous sedation.

Entry-site Divot

Tethering or divoting at the entry site is a rare occurrence and usually manifests as a dimple at the entry site during facial animation. This complication can easily be rectified by limited subcision using a Nokor™ or standard needle across the scar band.

POSTPROCEDURAL CARE

At the end of the procedure, the patient has no sutures, bandages, or drains of any kind unless a concurrent lifting procedure was performed that requires use of these ancillary measures. The patient is discharged after appropriate postanesthesia observance. Although some surgeons who perform fat transfer do not advocate immediate postoperative icing of transplanted regions given the risk of reducing fat-cell viability, we think that there is no compromise to the aesthetic result and recovery is expedited. We advocate intermittent icing for the first 48 to 72 hours postoperatively, which can be continued if the patient desires. Head elevation also reduces the extent of postoperative edema, but a restful night's sleep

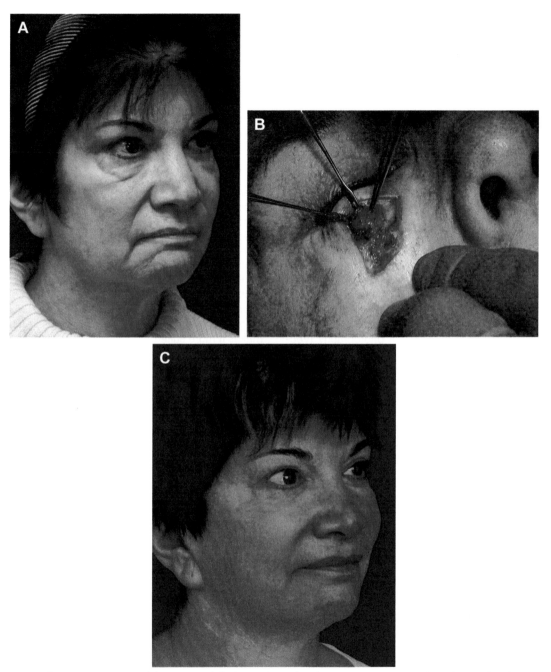

Fig. 6. (*A*) Preoperative view. (*B*) Excision of the lump through a discrete incision along the inferior orbital rim at the junction of the thin lower lid skin and the thicker cheek skin. (C) Postoperative view. (*From* Lam SM, Glasgold MJ, Glasgold RA. Complementary fat grafting. Philadelphia: Lippincott Williams & Wilkins, 2007; with permission.)

is of paramount importance and thus this is only stressed for the first several nights after surgery. Although heavy exercise, especially with increased intra-abdominal pressure and bending over, should be avoided, a light isometric weight-lifting regimen with one-half to one-third the typical weight and lighter cardiovascular exercise can be

undertaken, typically by the fourth or fifth postoperative day. In addition, salt intake should be limited because this assists in the resolution of postoperative edema.

Although postoperative care is simple and straightforward, management of postoperative expectations may be more involved. Patients may perceive that their faces appear too inflated for their liking in the first several postoperative weeks and regard this outcome as an unintended result. Although the expected course of recovery will have been explained in detail preoperatively, constant reassurance must be offered, with patients returning as often as necessary for encouragement and counsel. In addition, the ecchymosis and edema are often more pronounced in conjunction with a brow or face-lift and can be a social and professional encumbrance for a longer period of time. In addition, the fat harvesting sites are generally sore for the first several days to weeks after surgery.

CLINICAL RESULTS IN THE LITERATURE AND EVIDENCE

Improving the predictability and reliability of autologous fat grafting has been one of the primary interests. We assessed long-term (>1 year) volume changes after autologous fat grafting to the midface using three-dimensional photography (Vectra; Canfield) and found our average take to be 32% with an average injection volume of 10 mL in 1 side of the midface. The range of take was 10% to 88%.[11] With an average take of only about 3 mL and volume that was highly unpredictable only 20% of the patients thought that they needed a second procedure. This finding supports the idea that smaller volumes over larger areas with transitions into surrounding areas are desirable and produces an overall result that is better than using any individual site. It also made us reflect on our understanding of end points. Based on the aging theory of shadow patterns, the youthful effect is achieved by adding enough volume to a hollow to fill it and create a highlight, which implies that for any given hollow on the face there is a large range of volumes that will fill it. For example, filling a midface depression may be acceptable with volume takes of between 2 and 5 mL.

Hoping to improve the take of our autologous fat grafting we assessed different techniques of processing the fat.[12] Puregraft® is a membrane filtration system for processing fat developed by Cytori Therapeutics as part of the technology for isolating adipose-derived stem cells. We studied long-term take of midface fat transfers using this system and found an average take of 49% at 7 months. This percentage is a significant improvement compared with centrifuge processing. The Puregraft® processed fat has less free lipid content and contaminant blood and a higher volume of potentially viable fat.[13]

We also studied the effect of harvesting cannula design on the fat graft. We originally used a 4-mm keel–type cannula for harvesting. Recently, cheese grater–type cannulas were introduced. Using the Puregraft® system we were able to compare the fat obtained with each cannula type. The yield of injectable potentially viable fat from the cheese grater cannulas was significantly lower than from the keel, with a greater amount of free lipid content. For this reason we currently only recommend keel-type cannulas for harvesting.

SUMMARY

There is currently a major paradigm shift from excision-based surgery to strictly volume enhancement. As the perfect facial filler has not yet been found, development of synthetic facial injectables continues to advance at a remarkable pace. Just a few years ago, bovine collagen was the only US Food and Drug Administration (FDA)–approved synthetic filler. As the FDA proceeds with the approval process there are many choices. Each type of filler carries a specific characteristic that makes it more suited for a certain clinical application. The continuing changes in facial fillers offer the possibility of volume augmentation procedures with less downtime and without the need for harvesting fat.

A combined approach requiring judicious selection of lifting procedures and fat grafting tailored to each individual is advocated.[14] Whatever the outcome, it seems that fat grafting and facial volume enhancement represent the present and future of facial rejuvenation. We predict that volume enhancement will continue to play an increasing role as both a complementary procedure and as a stand-alone procedure in facial rejuvenation.

REFERENCES

1. Lam SM. A new paradigm for the aging face. Facial Plast Surg Clin North Am 2010;18(1):1–6.
2. Lam SM, Glasgold RA, Glasgold MJ. Fat harvesting techniques for facial fat transfer. Facial Plast Surg 2010;26(5):356–61.
3. Glasgold MJ, Lam SM, Glasgold RA. Complementary Fat Grafting. In: Papel I, editor. Facial Plastic and Reconstructive Surgery. 3rd edition. New York: Thieme; 2008.
4. Lam SM. Fat grafting: an alternative or adjunct to facelift surgery? Facial Plast Surg Clin North Am 2013;21(2):253–64.
5. Coleman SR. Structural fat grafts: the ideal filler? Clin Plast Surg 2001;28(1):111–9.
6. Lam S, Glasgold M, Glasgold R. Complementary Fat Grafting. Philadelphia: Lippincott, Williams & Wilkins; 2007.

7. Mendelson B, Wong CH. Changes in the facial skeleton with aging: implications and clinical applications in facial rejuvenation. Aesthetic Plast Surg 2012;36(4):753–60.

8. Massry GG, Azizzadeh B. Periorbital fat grafting. Facial Plast Surg 2013;29(1):46–57.

9. Mendelson BC, Muzaffar AR, Adams WP Jr. Surgical anatomy of the midcheek and malar mounds. Plast Reconstr Surg 2002;110(3):885–96 [discussion: 897–911].

10. Geissler PJ, Davis K, Roostaeian J, et al. Improving fat transfer viability: the role of aging, body mass index, and harvest site. Plast Reconstr Surg 2014; 134(2):227–32.

11. Meier JD, Glasgold RA, Glasgold MJ. 3D photography in the objective analysis of volume augmentation including fat augmentation and dermal fillers. Facial Plast Surg Clin North Am 2011;19(4):725–35, ix.

12. Botti G, Pascali M, Botti C, et al. A clinical trial in facial fat grafting: filtered and washed versus centrifuged fat. Plast Reconstr Surg 2011;127(6): 2464–73.

13. Gerth DJ, King B, Rabach L, et al. Long-term volumetric retention of autologous fat grafting processed with closed-membrane filtration. Aesthet Surg J 2014;34(7):985–94.

14. Lamb J. Volume rejuvenation of the face. Mo Med 2010;107(3):198–202.

Midface Volumization with Injectable Fillers

Marietta Tan, MD[a], Theda C. Kontis, MD[b],*

KEYWORDS

- Midface volume • Tear trough deformity • Hyaluronic acid • Calcium hydroxylapatite
- Poly-L-lactic acid • Polymethyl methacrylate • Midface injectable fillers

KEY POINTS

- Aging changes of the midface include loss of bony support, facial lipoatrophy, and descent of soft tissues.
- Restoration of midface volume can be achieved by the use of injectable filling agents.
- The improvement in lower lid and midface volume achieved with the use of filling agents can produce results lasting up to 2 years.
- Injection techniques in this region may vary and can include the use of needles or cannulas for product placement.
- Complications of soft tissue filler injections to the midface are generally mild and self-limiting.

INTRODUCTION

In recent years, our understanding of the changes associated with facial aging has improved. Volume deficit, rather than vertical descent or ptosis alone, is now appreciated as a critical component of facial aging. We understand volume loss in terms of bony remodeling of the craniofacial skeleton, lipoatrophy of the fat pads, and loss of skin and muscle tone.[1] In addition, the skin of the aging face loses volume and elasticity. In the midface and periorbital area, loss of volume results in a number of changes characteristic of the facial aging process. The tear trough and lid–cheek junction become more visible, and the malar region flattens and descends.

Our focus on facial rejuvenation has added the 3-dimensional idea of volume restoration to the traditional 2-dimensional process of surgically repositioning ptotic tissues. Volumizing the midface may be accomplished with either autologous fat or currently available filling materials. In the early 2000s, new classes of filling agents were developed that proved to be superior to collagen in both effect and duration of results. Many such filling materials have since gained tremendous popularity in the nonsurgical treatment of volume loss seen with facial aging. A number of filler materials, including hyaluronic acid (HA), calcium hydroxylapatite (CaHA), polymethyl methacrylate (PMMA) and poly-L-lactic acid (PLLA), are now available in the United States.[2]

TREATMENT GOALS

Given our current understanding of the central role of volume loss in facial aging, facial rejuvenation techniques have shifted away from treating wrinkles alone and toward increasing volume while shaping and sculpting the face. Injectable fillers can be used to restore volume and reduce the

Disclosures: Speaker's Bureau: Allergan, Inc (Irvine CA), Galderma Laboratories (Fort Worth, TX); Injection trainer: Galderma Laboratories (T.C. Kontis).
[a] Department of Otolaryngology-Head and Neck Surgery, Johns Hopkins University School of Medicine, 601 North Caroline Street, 6th Floor, Baltimore, MD 21287, USA; [b] Department of Otolaryngology-Head and Neck Surgery, Johns Hopkins Medical Institutions, 1838 Greene Tree Road, Suite 370, Baltimore, MD 21208, USA
* Corresponding author. Facial Plastic Surgicenter, Ltd, 1838 Greene Tree Road, Suite 370, Baltimore, MD 21208.
E-mail address: tckontis@aol.com

appearance of wrinkles and folds, thereby creating a more youthful appearance. Injectable fillers are especially useful in midface and periorbital rejuvenation, because many of the effects of aging in these areas are owing to volume depletion.

The specific goals of treatment must be ascertained for each individual patient. The selection of filler material and placement, as well as injection technique, must then be tailored for each patient, taking into account the specific anatomic changes observed in that individual, age and medical comorbidities, willingness for downtime, and cost.[3]

PRETREATMENT ASSESSMENT

The boundaries of the midface are the inferior orbital rim superiorly, the nasal sidewall medially, and the nasolabial fold inferiorly and along the course of the zygomaticus major muscle laterally (**Fig. 1**). Understanding of facial anatomy and of the contributions of different anatomic components to overall facial aging in each specific patient is critical in the selection and use of injection fillers. Careful assessment of each tissue layer of this region is paramount in determining treatments for facial rejuvenation, to obtain natural-looking results.

The lower lids and midface should be analyzed with the patient in a seated and upright position. Attention should be directed toward the degree of skeletonization of the lower lids, degree of orbital fat herniation, midface volume, and soft tissue ptosis. Fillers can be placed in the lower lid and/or the cheek to rejuvenate the midface, similar to the placement of autologous fat.

Lower Lid

The lower lid complex consists of skin, fat, and bone. In the lower lid, the tear trough refers to the depression extending from the medial canthus. It separates the lower eyelid from the cheek and is bound superiorly by the orbital fat pad. The tear trough ends approximately at the midpupillary line. Extending laterally from this point is an additional groove called the lid–cheek junction, which is roughly parallel to the infraorbital rim. The muscle components of both the tear trough and lid–cheek junction are fixed to bone; inferior descent of these structures is therefore minimal.[4] The tear trough and lid–cheek junction instead become more visible with age because of volume loss.[5] In addition, with aging, the central portion of the orbicularis-retaining ligament becomes more lax, resulting in inferior displacement of the orbital fat pads.[4] Herniation or pseudoherniation of the fat pad above produces lower lid "bags," deepens the tear trough, and further accentuates the trough by creating shadowing beneath. The inferior orbital rim becomes skeletonized and these changes produce the tear trough deformity.

The tear trough and lid–cheek junction are also defined by differences between the eyelid and cheek skin. The skin of the lower eyelid is thinner and more pigmented than that of the upper cheek; the upper cheek also has a thicker dermis and more underlying subcutaneous fat. With time, lid skin can become even more pigmented, increasing the contrast between the lid and the upper cheek.[6]

Evaluation of each of these components is critical before proceeding with lower lid volumization with injectable fillers. Ideal candidates have thick skin and are without large orbital fat pads. Patients with significant herniation of orbital fat may instead benefit more from surgery, because fillers alone may not eliminate adequately the transition between the protuberant fat pad and the concave tear trough.[7,8]

Midface

Evaluation of the midface for volumization should include assessment of both the soft tissue and bony components of the region. Fat in this area exists in several well-defined compartments in superficial and deep layers. With facial aging, there is volume depletion in these compartments. There is also ptosis and migration of the fat compartments.[9] As volume is lost and tissues descend, the malar bags become prominent owing to the tethering of the zygomaticocutaneous ligament. The skin also becomes ptotic. In addition, bone remodeling of the midface and orbit contributes to the change in appearance of the overlying soft tissues.[10] As a result of these changes, the full "apple cheeks" of youth become deflated. Ideal candidates for midface volume restoration have a

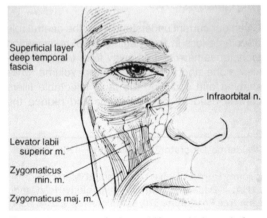

Fig. 1. Anatomy of the midface. (*Adapted from* Schwarcz RM, Kotlus B. Complications of lower blepharoplasty and midface lifting. Clin Plast Surg 2015;42(1):63–71; with permission.)

Superficial layer deep temporal fascia

Infraorbital n.

Levator labii superior m.

Zygomaticus min. m.

Zygomaticus maj. m.

minimal to moderate tear trough deformity and diminished volume in the cheeks, with minimal to moderate soft tissue descent.

PRODUCT SELECTION
Lower Lid

Volume restoration of the tear trough with filler materials is a difficult technique to master and should only be performed by well-trained practitioners. The lower lid region may be particularly difficult to inject, given its thin skin and its proximity to the orbital and malar fat pads. HA products are widely used in this area given their safety profiles, low allergic potential, and relative ease of injection. Furthermore, HA fillers can be dissolved with hyaluronidase, another advantage when treating this unforgiving region of the face.

In one author's opinion (T.K.), only 2 Food and Drug Administration (FDA)-approved HA fillers — Restylane (Galderma Laboratories, Fort Worth, TX) and Belotero (Merz Aesthetics, Greensboro, NC) — are appropriate fillers to use in this region. The thin, syruplike nature of Juvederm combined with the motion of the orbicularis muscle results in pooling of the product over time. Restylane, however, has a more ideal consistency for placement in the lower lids (**Fig. 2**), although superficial placement or migration of the product may result in a bluish hue under the skin (**Fig. 3**). This discoloration is referred to as the Tyndall effect, which is believed to result from the refraction of blue light by the uniformly sized Restylane particles.[11] Occasionally, hyaluronidase injections are necessary to correct this deformity by rapid enzymatic degradation of the product.

Belotero, on the other hand, is manufactured by a different process (CPM technology), which creates a polydensified matrix. This produces a product with more uniform particle size than Restylane, which allows it to spread more easily. It may therefore be injected more superficially and is less likely to result in the Tyndall effect (**Fig. 4**).[11] Unlike Restylane, Belotero does not have lidocaine added to the product. Because of its hydrophilic nature, undiluted Belotero can result in significant edema of the lower lids; dilution of the product by the addition of lidocaine just before injection is therefore suggested.

Midface

Volumization of the malar region is technically simple, and a variety of fillers are appropriate for this region. HA, CaHA, PLLA, and PMMA have all been used to augment the midface with good results. However, only 1 filler, the HA product Juvederm Voluma (Allergan, Irvine, CA), has been FDA approved to treat this region.

Hyaluronic acid

HA is a naturally occurring polysaccharide found in the skin, cartilage, synovial joint fluid, and other connective tissues and is identical in structure across all mammalian species.[12] It is an ideal filler because it is biodegradable and nonimmunogenic. There are many HA filler products available; they differ in their degree of cross-linking, gel consistency, and concentration. They have been shown to have good safety profiles and excellent outcomes (**Fig. 5**).[2]

Injection of HA fillers may be performed using 27- or 30-gauge needles. Alternatively, cannulas may also be used. This author (T.K.) prefers to use an injection of 1% xylocaine with 1:100,000 epinephrine at the needle entry site. The cannula is then inserted through a control hole made with a 25-gauge needle. The product is then feathered in the deep subcutaneous tissue or preperiosteal plane.

Juvederm Voluma is a newer filling material that received FDA approval in late 2013 for midface volumization.[13] The pivotal study by Jones and Murphy[14] showed it was safe and effective for up to 2 years. The injection technique for Voluma begins with injections in the upper outer quadrant, proceeding inferomedially to give volume to the cheek.

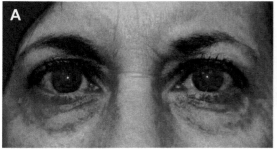
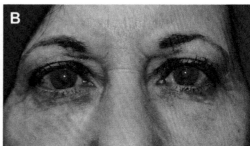

Fig. 2. Before (A) and after (B) injection of Restylane to the tear trough and infraorbital rim.

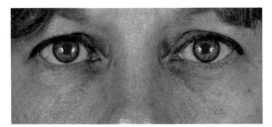

Fig. 3. Tyndall effect: injected product appears blue when placed too superficially under the skin.

Calcium hydroxylapatite

Radiesse (Merz Aesthetics) is composed of spheres of CaHA in an aqueous gel carrier. Unlike HA, Radiesse works as a volumizer by stimulating production of collagen; the microspheres act as a scaffold for the newly formed collagen. The carrier gel is resorbed within several weeks after injection, and the CaHA itself slowly degrades over time and is excreted by the body. Like HA, CaHA is nonimmunogenic and biodegradable, with a favorable safety profile.[2] Radiesse works well to fill the midface because it has a high lift capacity and results may persist for about a year (**Fig. 6**).

CaHA can be placed in the midface with either a cannula or a needle, in a manner similar to injection of HA products.[15] Radiesse premixed with lidocaine is not available commercially, although the product received FDA approval in 2009 for the addition of lidocaine before injection. The product should be injected into the subdermal or preperiosteal plane.

Polymethyl methacrylate

PMMA (Artefill, Suneva Medical, San Diego, CA) may also be used for midface volumization. It is a permanent filler and is composed of microspheres of PMMA suspended in a matrix of bovine collagen and lidocaine. After injection, volume is initially provided by the collagen gel. The collagen is resorbed by the body over 1 to 3 months, while the PMMA becomes encapsulated with connective tissue during this time. The PMMA microspheres are not degraded or excreted by the body; results, therefore, are permanent and cannot be reversed. Despite being a nonabsorbable implant, the safety profile of PMMA is similar to that of HA or CaHA fillers.[2]

Owing to the bovine-based carrier gel, skin testing must be performed 1 month before injection to rule out an allergic reaction. Injection of the product into the midface may be performed using either a needle or cannula into the subdermal or preperiosteal plane. Care must be taken to place the product symmetrically and to undercorrect.

Poly-L-lactic acid

PLLA (Sculptra, Galderma Laboratories) is another useful product to augment the malar region,[16] which consists of lyophilized crystals of PLLA that must be rehydrated by in the addition of water. PLLA is a synthetic polymer that stimulates collagen production by causing a foreign body reaction and dermal fibrosis. It is biodegradable, although the product may persist for a variable period of time, up to several years.[2] Injections should be performed over several sessions at 6-week intervals for optimal facial volumization (**Fig. 7**). The product should be placed in the subdermal plane. Patients should be counseled that final results can take months to achieve.

INJECTION PROCEDURE

Before injection of the midface, photographs are taken to highlight the lower lids and cheeks. A three-quarter view of the face shows the contours of the cheeks and outlines the cheek prominence (see **Fig. 7**). Informed consent must be obtained before any injection procedure and should include a discussion of the risks of vascular injury, asymmetry, bruising, lumpiness, and the need for subsequent touch-up treatments.

Lower Lid

Injection of the lower lids should be performed with the patient in an upright position. Per patient and physician preference, topical anesthetic cream

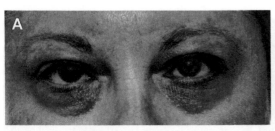
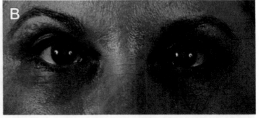

Fig. 4. Before (*A*) and after (*B*) injection of Belotero into the lower lids and tear trough. (The patient has also undergone an upper lid blepharoplasty. She initially had Restylane placed, which migrated superficially over several years and the Tyndall deformity resulted. Product was dissolved with hyaluronidase and Belotero placed 2 weeks later.)

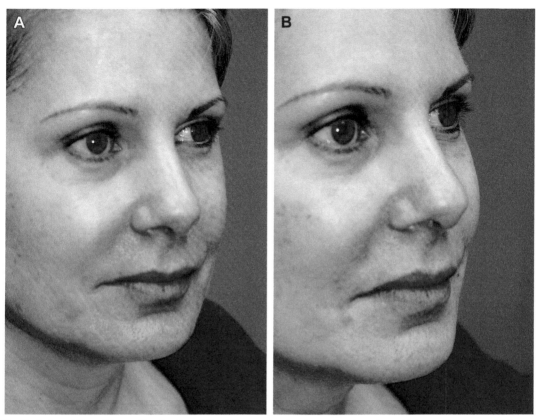

Fig. 5. Before (*A*) and immediately after (*B*) midface volumization using Juvederm Voluma (1 mL per side).

can be applied to the lower lids before the injection procedure. However, this is not a painful area to inject, and patients often tolerate injection of this area without topical numbing.

Most injectors find that deep injection of HA along the bony orbital rim is the ideal place for injection. Superficial injections increase bruising and risk of the Tyndall effect. Small aliquots (0.1–0.2 mL) are placed and massaged into place. Change in orbital gaze position alters the position of the filling material, so having the patient open their eyes and look up aids in correct placement.

The use of cannulas has become increasing common for use in augmenting the tear trough region to lessen the risk of vascular injury. When using a cannula, a "control hole" must first be created in the midcheek region. This author (T.K.) prefers to use a small injection of 1% xylocaine with 1:100,000 epinephrine before creating the entry site with a 25-gauge needle. Using a

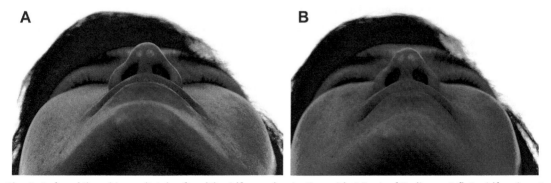

Fig. 6. Before (*A*) and immediately after (*B*) midface volumization with 1.5 mL of Radiesse. A flat midface is not uncommon in the Asian population and augmentation in this region can soften the midface.

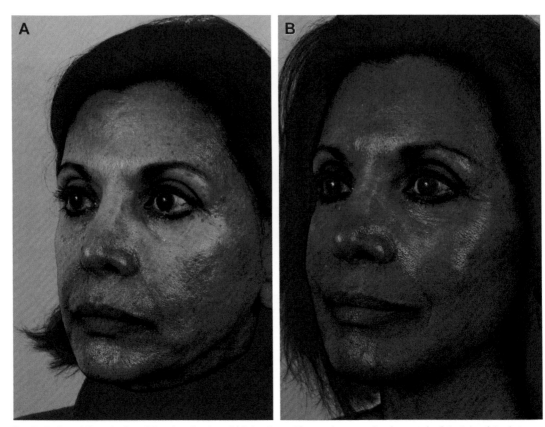

Fig. 7. Before (*A*) and after (*B*) poly-L-lactic acid injections. The patient received a total of 6 vials of Sculptra.

27-gauge cannula inserted through this entry point, filler is placed deeply along the infraorbital rim, in a method not unlike autologous fat placement, and then gently pressed into place to reduce lumpiness and to smooth contours.

Midface

Before the introduction of Juvederm Voluma, practitioners placed fillers (an "off-label" use) in the cheeks and malar prominence in a manner they thought would be aesthetically pleasing. A variety of products including HA,[17] CaHA, PLLA, and occasionally PMMA[18] were placed either transcutaneously or via the buccal sulcus. No reports of increased risk of infection have been published using the transoral route. However, more recent studies of midface volumization with filler materials have added to our understanding of patient assessment and ideal product placement.

Hinderer's lines were used to delineate the location on maximal cheek prominence (**Fig. 8**).[19] Dr Ulrich Hinderer was a plastic surgeon practicing in Madrid, Spain, who developed silicone malar shell implants for the correction of a flat midface and published his work in 1975. A man before his time, Hinderer expressed surprise that there was

so little attention placed on the zygomatic region. He stated that, because persons are generally viewed in oblique profile and "high cheekbones" contribute to a youthful oval face, augmentation of the zygomatic region would enhance beauty. He described 2 lines: one drawn from the lateral canthus to the lateral oral commissure and the other from the tragus to the nasal ala. The majority of his implant should ideally be placed in the upper–outer quadrant. The Voluma studies defined the quadrants divided by Hinderer's lines into 3 subsegments: the zygomaticomalar, anteromedial, and submalar regions.[14]

The injection technique in this region has not been well-defined until recently when studies of Juvederm Voluma standardized techniques for this region. Injections are initiated laterally in a depot technique, in a region similar to the location of Hinderer's malar shell. Filler product is generally placed deeply.

POSTPROCEDURE CARE
Lower Lid

After treatment, patients are asked to use cold compresses on their lower lids for the first day and to refrain from exercise until any bruises resolve.

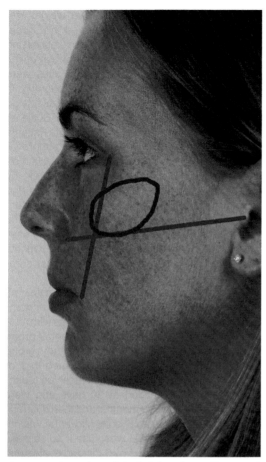

Fig. 8. Hinderer's lines (*black*) define the midface quadrants. The maximal cheek volume lies in the upper–outer or zygomatico–malar region (*blue*) and is the region targeted for volume enhancement of the midface.

Once the swelling subsides, a touch-up treatment may be required, so it is important to reassess these patients in approximately 2 weeks after initial injection. If the patient notes lumpiness, a warm compress should be placed over the lid for 20 minutes while applying firm but gentle pressure. This may help to flatten lumps and minor irregularities.

Midface

Patients who have undergone midface injection with HA, CaHA, and PMMA have very few postinjection sequelae. The use of ice packs aids with any bruising or swelling that develops. For those patients who have undergone PLLA injections, we advise facial massage for 5 minutes a day, 5 times a day, for the next 5 days.

COMPLICATIONS

Complications of filler injections to the face are generally mild and self-resolving. The most common complications are bruising, edema, and pain or tenderness.[20] The use of cold compresses or ice packs may help to reduce these complications. Lumpiness or asymmetry are also possible and may be treated with massage and warm compresses.

Other adverse events include allergic reactions to the filler material, infections, and granulomas. True immunoglobulin E-mediated immune reactions (type I hypersensitivity) are rare. For example, hypersensitivity to HA occurs in approximately 1 in 5000 cases.[11] Type I hypersensitivity may result in local or generalized facial edema, which can be treated with antihistamines or oral steroids. Delayed hypersensitivity reactions are also possible and result in induration and erythema days to weeks after injection.[21] Infection at the site of injection are rare and may be treated with either antibiotics or antivirals, depending on the type of infection.[11] Foreign body granulomas may occur with permanent fillers but are uncommon with HA products. These painless nodules typically develop between 6 and 24 months after injection and can persist for years. They are usually effectively treated with intralesional or oral steroids.[22]

The most serious complication of injectable fillers is vascular compromise leading to skin necrosis. Vascular compromise may result from direct injury to vessels during injection, external compression of vessels by filler material, or intraluminal injection of product. If vascular injury goes unnoticed or untreated, necrosis of the tissues supplied by the affected vessel may result. The risk of vascular injury may be reduced, but not eliminated, by the use of blunt cannulas instead of needles. The earliest sign of potential vascular compromise is blanching at the site of injection and typically occurs at the time of injection. Further injection should be stopped. The area should then be treated with massage and warm compresses. Topical nitroglycerin paste should also be applied to the region for further vasodilation, and aspirin should be administered. Consider hyaluronidase injections no matter which product was being used. The patient should be closely monitored to assess progress of the injury.[23]

Lower Lid

Volume replacement in the lower lids can be challenging for the injector, regardless of their skill level. Bruising, swelling, globe motion, and skin thinness contribute to the difficulty in achieving a perfect result.

As previously noted, a possible complication of lower lid injections is the Tyndall effect, or a bluish hue underneath the skin resulting from refraction of light by HA filler particles. The Tyndall effect is more likely if filler material is injected too superficially. Injection deep to the orbicularis oculi muscle reduces the risk of discoloration.[3] Alternatively, Belotero is less likely to result in the Tyndall effect even when injected superficially owing to its unique polydensified matrix consistency. The Tyndall effect may be treated by dissolving the HA product with hyaluronidase.

Reports of serious complications like blindness have been described with periorbital injections, but such events are extremely rare.[24] Injection of filler directly into a distal branch of the ophthalmic artery (including the dorsal nasal artery and angular artery of the nose) can result in retrograde flow of the past the origin of the central retinal artery. Anterograde flow can then propel the filler into the retinal artery, resulting in permanent blindness.[25] As with other vascular events, the risk of intraarterial injection is decreased by the use of blunt cannulas. The risk of blindness is also minimized by injecting slowly and with minimal pressure.[26]

Midface

Complications of midface augmentation are generally mild and self-limiting. The most common complications of filler injections to the malar region include bruising, edema, lumpiness, and asymmetry. There are no major end vessels in this region, so injection of fillers in this area is relatively safe. This author (T.K.) finds the most difficult aspect of malar augmentation with fillers to be obtaining exact symmetry. Because some patients have subtle facial asymmetries, injections must be placed for symmetry and different amounts of filler material may be required from one side to the other.

OUTCOMES

In clinical trials of facial fillers, the nasolabial folds have been the most commonly addressed area of the face.[2] Many descriptive and qualitative studies have been published that assess the use of fillers for lower lid and midface volumization, but few randomized, controlled trials exist.[26–28] Given this dearth of clinical trials, commercially available fillers are generally FDA-approved only for the treatment of facial folds and wrinkles, such as the nasolabial folds, or human immunodeficiency virus (HIV)-related facial lipoatrophy. However, injectable fillers are frequently used for volumization of the lower lid and midface regions in an "off-label" fashion.

Only 1 filler available in the United States, Juvederm Voluma, has been granted FDA approval specifically to treat age-related midface volume loss. Juvederm Voluma is an HA gel with a mixture of low- and high-molecular-weight HA. The first study of Voluma, performed in Europe, was an open-label, nonrandomized trial assessing the safety profile, benefit, and ease of use of the product. Seventy patients across 15 sites were included. Injections were performed primarily in the malar region (59%). Patients were evaluated using the 5-point Facial Volume Loss Scale at baseline and at day 14 after treatment. Patients were also rated on the Global Aesthetic Improvement Scale (GAIS) at day 14. The mean Facial Volume Loss Scale score declined significantly by day 14. Using the GAIS, 88% of physicians and 76% of patients rated their level of improvement as much improved or very much improved. The vast majority of physicians rated Voluma as easy to use. Adverse events occurred in 24 patients and were transient; bruising was the most common adverse event.[29]

FDA approval was granted for Juvederm Voluma after the completion of a single-blinded, randomized controlled clinical trial of 282 patients with midface volume loss. The no-treatment control group included 47 patients, whereas the study group included 235 patients, who were treated in 1 or more of midface regions. Patients received touch-up treatments as needed at 30 days and were seen again at 1 month, 3 months, and then quarterly for 2 years. The validated 6-point Mid-Face Volume Deficit Scale (MFVDS) was used to assess improvement at 6 months by 2 blinded evaluators. Improvement of 1 point or more on the MFVDS was achieved at 6 months by 85.6% of patients, with a significant difference between the control and treatment groups. On the GAIS, 82.2% of investigators and 92.8% of patients rated midface volume as improved or much improved at 6 months. Minimal adverse events were reported and included injection site tenderness, swelling, firmness, or lumpiness. Most adverse events resolved within 2 weeks or less.[14]

An additional open-label trial of Juvederm Voluma has since been completed. In a 24-month Australian trial, 103 patients underwent Voluma injections to the malar region. Subjects were evaluated at week 8, week 78, and month 24 using the MFVDS and GAIS. At week 8, 96% of patients achieved an improvement of 1 point or more on both MFVDS and GAIS ratings. A total of 72 subjects completed the 24-month study; of these, 45 did not require supplementary Voluma at week 78. At the completion of the study, 96% of those 45 patients who had not required touch-up treatments had retained improvement on MFVDS assessment. GAIS evaluation demonstrated continued improvement in 82% and 91% when rated by subjects and physicians, respectively.[30]

Other HA fillers that have been evaluated for volumization in the midface in open-label trials include Restylane SubQ (Medicis Aesthetics) and Perlane-L (Medicis Aesthetics). Restylane SubQ is a large-particle, stabilized HA gel designed for injection in the subcutaneous and supraperiosteal planes to restore volume loss and define facial contours. A 12-month, open-label study was performed to assess the safety and efficacy of the product for cheek and chin augmentation. Fifty-seven patients underwent injection, for a total of 98 cheeks treated. Patients were evaluated using the GAIS at several intervals up to 12 months. This study did not distinguish between those treated in for cheek versus chin augmentation, but overall patients and investigators noted at least some improvement at treated sites in 91% and 96% at 6 months, respectively. By 12 months, response rates had fallen to 58% and 53% of subjects, respectively. Treatment-related adverse events included local reactions, induration, and implant mobility.[17]

Perlane-L is another large-particle HA, premixed with 0.3% lidocaine. Its effectiveness in volumizing and contouring the midface was evaluated in an open-label Canadian study. This 24-week trial included 40 patients who were rated at weeks 8 and 24 using the validated 4-point Medicis Midface Volume Scale and the GAIS. Improvement of at least 1 point on the Medicis Midface Volume Scale was noted in 97.5% and 90.0% at week 8, as rated by blinded evaluators and subjects, respectively. At week 24, continued improvement was noted in 90.0% and 82.5% of subjects, respectively. GAIS assessments showed improvement in 95.0% to 100.0% of subjects throughout the study period. Mild adverse events, including bruising, swelling, and pain, were reported, but had all resolved by week 24.[31]

Several fillers have been studied for their efficacy in treating HIV-related facial lipoatrophy. The use of Radiesse (CaHA) for augmentation in HIV lipoatrophy was examined in an 18-month open-label trial. One hundred subjects underwent injection of Radiesse into the cheek (typically submalar) regions. GAIS assessments demonstrated improvement in 100% of patients at 3 months and in 91% at 18 months. Treatment-related adverse events were generally mild and included bruising, swelling, redness, and pain.[32]

Injectable PLLA received FDA approval for treatment of HIV-associated lipoatrophy in 2004. Its efficacy and safety were first investigated in England in a 24-week, open-label, randomized study of 30 patients. Immediate versus delayed treatments were studied. The immediate group received injections into the deep dermis overlying the buccal fat pad on day 1 and weeks 2 and 4, whereas the

delayed group received injections at weeks 12, 14, and 16. Patients were assessed using visual analog scales as well as anxiety and depression scales. At week 12, the immediate treatment group had significantly better visual analog, anxiety, and depression scores than the delayed group; these improvements persisted through the end of the study period. No serious adverse events were reported.[33] These subjects were later reevaluated for long-term safety and efficacy. A sustained improvement in visual analog scales was seen after a minimum of 18 months after last injection. Delayed treatment-related adverse events included nodularity, but were not severe.[34]

Last, PMMA (Artefill) has been evaluated for safety and efficacy in malar augmentation for age-related lipoatrophy in a 12-month, open-label pilot study in Canada. A total of 24 patients with mild to moderate lipoatrophy underwent injection of Artefill in the supraperiosteal layer of the malar region, with touch-up injections at weeks 4 and 6. GAIS scores demonstrated that 95.8% of subjects were improved or very much improved, and malar lipoatrophy grades were significantly improved from baseline at 1 year after injection. There were no reported adverse events in this study.[18]

SUMMARY

The contribution of volume loss to facial aging is now more greatly appreciated, and we now consider the 3-dimensional changes of volume in addition to the 2-dimensional changes of ptosis that we have traditionally associated with aging. Volume loss occurs in all tissue compartments of the face, including skin, muscle, fat, and bone. Over the past decade, the popularity of injectable fillers has grown tremendously. Volumization of the lower lid and midface with fillers is fairly straightforward with few side effects, and it offers a number of advantages over surgical rejuvenation procedures when performed correctly and in the right patient. Clinicians must have knowledge of the available fillers and of facial anatomy, to minimize the risk of complications resulting from injection. Few randomized controlled trials have been conducted evaluating the use of injectable fillers in volumization, but available products have been used safely and effectively in an "off-label" fashion for many years. Many opportunities clearly exist for further research in these areas.

REFERENCES

1. Fitzgerald R, Vleggaar D. Facial volume restoration of the aging face with poly-L-lactic acid. Dermatol Ther 2011;24:2–27.

2. Kontis TC. Contemporary review of injectable facial fillers. JAMA Facial Plast Surg 2013;15(1):58–64.

3. Pontius AT, Chaiet SR, Williams EF 3rd. Midface injectable fillers: have they replaced midface surgery? Facial Plast Surg Clin North Am 2013;21(2):229–39.

4. Haddock NT, Saadeh PB, Boutros S, et al. The tear trough and lid/cheek junction: anatomy and implications for surgical correction. Plast Reconstr Surg 2009;123(4):1332–40.

5. Lambros V. Models of facial aging and implications for treatment. Clin Plast Surg 2008;35(3):319–27.

6. Lambros VS. Hyaluronic acid injections for correction of the tear trough deformity. Plast Reconstr Surg 2007; 120(6 Suppl):74S–80S.

7. Hirmand H. Anatomy and nonsurgical correction of the tear trough deformity. Plast Reconstr Surg 2010;125(2):699–708.

8. Stutman RL, Codner MA. Tear trough deformity: review of anatomy and treatment options. Aesthet Surg J 2012;32(4):426–40.

9. Gierloff M, Stöhring C, Buder T, et al. Aging changes of the midfacial fat compartments: a computed tomographic study. Plast Reconstr Surg 2012;129(1):263–73.

10. Shaw RB Jr, Katzel EB, Koltz PF, et al. Aging of the facial skeleton: aesthetic implications and rejuvenation strategies. Plast Reconstr Surg 2011;127(1):374–83.

11. Jones D. Volumizing the face with soft tissue fillers. Clin Plast Surg 2011;38(3):379–90.

12. Rohrich RJ, Ghavami A, Crosby MA. The role of hyaluronic acid fillers (Restylane) in facial cosmetic surgery: review and technical considerations. Plast Reconstr Surg 2007;120(6 Suppl):41S–54S.

13. Philipp-Dormston W, Eccleston D, DeBoulle K, et al. A prospective, observational study of the volumizing effect of open-label aesthetic use of Juvederm Voluma with Lidocaine in midface area. J Cosmet Laser Ther 2014;16:171–9.

14. Jones D, Murphy DK. Volumizing Hyaluronic acid filler for midface volume deficit: 2-year results from a pivotal single-blind randomized controlled study. Dermatol Surg 2013;39:1602–12.

15. Gravier MH, Bass LS, Busso M, et al. Calcium hydroxylapatite (Radiesse) for correction of the mid- and lower face: consensus recommendations. Plast Reconstr Surg 2007;120(6 Suppl):55S–66S.

16. Vleggaar D, Fitzgerald R, Lorenc P, et al. Consensus recommendations on the use of injectable poly-L-lactic acid for facial and nonfacial volumization. J Drugs Dermatol 2014;13(Suppl 4):s44–51.

17. DeLorenzi C, Weinberg M, Solish N, et al. The long-term efficacy and safety of a subcutaneously injected large-particle stabilized hyaluronic acid-based gel of nonanimal origin in esthetic facial contouring. Dermatol Surg 2009;35(Suppl 1):313–21.

18. Mills DC, Camp S, Mosser S, et al. Malar augmentation with a polymethylmethacrylate-enhanced filler: assessment of a 12-month open-label pilot study. Aesthet Surg J 2013;33(3):421–30.

19. Hinderer UT. Malar implants for the improvement of the facial appearance. Plast Reconstr Surg 1975; 56(2):157–65.

20. Glogau RG, Kane MA. Effect of injection techniques on the rate of local adverse events in patients implanted with nonanimal hyaluronic acid gel dermal fillers. Dermatol Surg 2008;34(Suppl 1):S105–9.

21. Funt D, Pavicic T. Dermal fillers in aesthetics: an overview of adverse events and treatment approaches. Clin Cosmet Investig Dermatol 2013;6:295–316.

22. Weinberg MJ, Solish N. Complications of hyaluronic acid fillers. Facial Plast Surg 2009;25(5):324–8.

23. DeLorenzi C. Complications of injectable fillers, part 2: vascular complications. Aesthet Surg J 2014;34(4): 584–600.

24. Ozturk CN, Li Y, Tung R, et al. Complications following injection of soft-tissue fillers. Aesthet Surg J 2013;33(6):862–77.

25. Coleman SR. Avoidance of arterial occlusion from injection of soft tissue fillers. Aesthet Surg J 2002; 22(6):555–7.

26. Kane MA. Treatment of tear trough deformity and lower lid bowing with injectable hyaluronic acid. Aesthetic Plast Surg 2005;29(5):363–7.

27. Morley AM, Malhotra R. Use of hyaluronic acid filler for tear-trough rejuvenation as an alternative to lower eyelid surgery. Ophthal Plast Reconstr Surg 2011;27(2):69–73.

28. Viana GA, Osaki MH, Cariello AJ, et al. Treatment of the tear trough deformity with hyaluronic acid. Aesthet Surg J 2011;31(2):225–31.

29. Hoffmann K, Juvéderm Voluma Study Investigators Group. Volumizing effects of a smooth, highly cohesive, viscous 20-mg/mL hyaluronic acid volumizing filler: prospective European study. BMC Dermatol 2009;9:9.

30. Callan P, Goodman GJ, Carlisle I, et al. Efficacy and safety of a hyaluronic acid filler in subjects treated for correction of midface volume deficiency: a 24 month study. Clin Cosmet Investig Dermatol 2013;6:81–9.

31. Bertucci V, Lin X, Axford-Gatley RA, et al. Safety and effectiveness of large gel particle hyaluronic acid with lidocaine for correction of midface volume loss. Dermatol Surg 2013;39(11):1621–9.

32. Silvers SL, Eviatar JA, Echavez MI, et al. Prospective, open-label, 18-month trial of calcium hydroxylapatite (Radiesse) for facial soft-tissue augmentation in patients with human immunodeficiency virus-associated lipoatrophy: one-year durability. Plast Reconstr Surg 2006; 118(3 Suppl):34S–45S.

33. Moyle GJ, Lysakova L, Brown S, et al. A randomized open-label study of immediate versus delayed poly-lactic acid injections for the cosmetic management of facial lipoatrophy in persons with HIV infection. HIV Med 2004;5(2):82–7.

34. Moyle GJ, Brown S, Lysakova L, et al. Long-term safety and efficacy of poly-L-lactic acid in the treatment of HIV-related facial lipoatrophy. HIV Med 2006;7(3):181–5.

The Role of Neurotoxins in the Periorbital and Midfacial Areas

Benjamin P. Erickson, MD[a], Wendy W. Lee, MD[b],
Joel Cohen, MD[c], Lisa D. Grunebaum, MD[d],*

KEYWORDS

- Botulinum toxin • Neurotoxin • Facial rhytids • AbobotulinumtoxinA • IncobotulinumtoxinA
- OnabotulinumtoxinA • RimabotulinumtoxinB

KEY POINTS

- Three neurotoxin formulations are approved for cosmetic use in the United States: onabotulinumtoxinA (Botox), abobotulinumtoxinA (Dysport), and incobotulinumtoxinA (Xeomin).
- Selection is dictated by injector and patient preference, patient history, and the presence of allergies, among other considerations.
- No 2 toxins are exactly the same unit for unit, and there is no universally accepted formula for unit conversion.
- Complications of botulinum neurotoxin injection, such as eyelid ptosis, brow ptosis, and double vision, can be reduced with appropriate reconstitution and injection techniques.
- The trend has been toward an individualized, sculpted approach that preserves baseline facial animation and accounts for the gender, ethnicity, individual preference, and professional needs.

 Videos of female and male glabellar injections and lateral canthal line injection accompany this article at http://www.facialplastic.theclinics.com/

INTRODUCTION

The concept of therapeutic botulinum toxin (BoNT) injection was ushered in by Dr Allen Scott's landmark study in the late 1970s, which demonstrated safety and efficacy for the treatment of adult strabismus.[1] The US Food and Drug Administration (FDA) approved the first commercial BoNT formulation, onabotulinumtoxinA, for the treatment of strabismus and blepharospasm in 1989. After Carruthers and Carruthers[2] first recognized the dramatic reduction of glabellar rhytids in patients treated for essential for blepharospasm, however, it took more than a decade for the FDA to extend approval to esthetic indications, long after the toxin was already popularized for cosmetic use.

Since the approval of cosmetic Botox in 2002, the number of annual treatments has skyrocketed, making BoNT injections the top nonsurgical esthetic enhancement worldwide for more than a decade. Facial injections were the single most common cosmetic procedure in 2011, accounting for 41% of all esthetic interventions performed in the United States.[3] According to 2013 data from the American Society of Plastic Surgeons, 6.3 million cosmetic BoNT A injections were performed, nearly 3 times the number of dermal filler treatments.[4] Market

[a] Bascom Palmer Eye Institute, University of Miami Miller School of Medicine, 900 NW 17th Street, Miami, FL 33136, USA; [b] Department of Clinical Ophthalmology and Dermatology Oculofacial Plastic & Reconstructive Surgery, Orbit and Oncology, Bascom Palmer Eye Institute, University of Miami Miller School of Medicine, 900 NW 17th Street, Miami, FL 33136, USA; [c] AboutSkin Dermatology, 499 East Hamden Avenue, Suite 450, Englewood, CO 80113, USA; [d] Division of Facial Plastic and Reconstructive Surgery, Department of Otolaryngology and Dermatology, University of Miami Miller School of Medicine, 900 NW 17th Street, Miami, FL 33136, USA
* Corresponding author. Facial Plastic Surgery, 1150 Northwest 14th Street, Miami, FL 33136.
E-mail address: lgrunebaum@med.miami.edu

Facial Plast Surg Clin N Am 23 (2015) 243–255
http://dx.doi.org/10.1016/j.fsc.2015.01.010
1064-7406/15/$ – see front matter © 2015 Elsevier Inc. All rights reserved.

expansion continues at an impressive rate, particularly among men. The number of males seeking cosmetic injections has grown by 268% since 2000.[3] Satisfaction and rates of return for repeat injections are very high, making it both an excellent source of practice revenue and an effective way of introducing patients to other cosmetic treatments.

Seven distinct serotypes of BoNT (A–G) have been isolated from different strains of *Clostridium botulinum*.[5–7] Only BoNT-A and BoNT-B, which function exclusively in cholinergic neurons, have been approved for clinical use.[5] There are currently 4 neurotoxin formulations available for injection in the United States: onabotulinumtoxinA (onaBoNT-A, Botox, Allergan, Inc, Irvine, CA), abobotulinumtoxinA (aboBoNT-A, Dysport, Galderma Laboratories, L.P., Fort Worth, TX), incobotulinumtoxinA (incoBoNT-A, Xeomin, Merz Pharmaceuticals, L.L.C., Greensboro, NC), and rimabotulinumtoxinB (rimaBoNT-B, Myobloc, Solstice Neurosciences, Inc, San Francisco, CA). All 3 BoNT-A preparations are approved for the correction of moderate-to-severe glabellar lines but only onaBoNT-A is approved for lateral canthal lines; all other uses remain off label.[8]

In nature, BoNT consists of a 150-kDa core. With the exception of incoBoNT-A, this core is surrounded by varying amounts of nontoxic complexing proteins.[9] These proteins are thought to stabilize the neurotoxin, protecting it from pH and temperature fluctuations as well as lytic enzymes.[10] Although these accessory proteins confer an obvious advantage to the *Clostridial* bacillus during gastrointestinal transit, the benefits are less clear for therapeutic use. In fact, there is mounting evidence that the presence of complexing proteins merely increases neurotoxin antigenicity without prolonging product shelf life.[11] Accordingly, most manufacturers have worked to reduce the foreign protein load present in each unit of BoNT.

BoNT functions at the level of the neuromuscular junction by blocking acetylcholine release, thus decreasing contraction of the motor unit. It is taken up in the presynaptic terminal via receptor-mediated endocytosis.[9] In the acidic environment of the endosome, a disulfide bond is cleaved, separating the core protein into heavy and light chains, which are the active moieties.[5,9,12] By irreversibly inhibiting components of the SNARE complex, BoNT prevents nontoxic exocytosis; BoNT-A cleaves SNAP-25, whereas BoNT-B cleaves synaptobrevin.[5,13]

With ongoing turnover at the neuromuscular junction, however, contractile function begins to return after several weeks, and usually attains pretreatment strength by 6 months.[13] From a cosmetic and therapeutic standpoint, treatments generally remain effective for 3 to 4 months, and there is no evidence of tachyphylaxis in the majority of patients.[9,14]

TREATMENT GOALS

The superficial facial mimetic muscles insert directly onto the undersurface of the skin; repetitive contraction therefore causes characteristic furrows (rhytids) to form perpendicular to the direction of contraction. Although injection of BoNT does not eliminate static wrinkling, it can reduce dramatically the appearance of hyperdynamic lines in the midface and periocular region via selective chemodenervation.

Since the introduction of cosmetic Botox, treatment goals and therapeutic endpoints have continued to evolve. The trend has been away from a one-size-fits-all 'frozen' appearance, and toward a more subtle, individualized approach. It is important to account for the gender, ethnicity, individual preference, and professional needs of each patient. With careful appraisal of each patient's anatomy, injection can produce a harmonious appearance in which facial animation is preserved. By selectively targeting depressors in preference to elevators, modest lifting and sculpting can also be achieved.

Synergies can be obtained by combining BoNT injection with dermal fillers, cutaneous lasers, retinoids, and facial plastic surgery.[12] Because most rhytids have both static and dynamic contributions, the optimal approach often combines neurotoxin and dermal filler injections. A number of studies report improved patient satisfaction and more durable results when BoNT and hyaluronic acid treatments are administered in tandem.[15,16]

PREOPERATIVE PLANNING AND PREPARATION
Selecting a Product

Three different formulations of BoNT-A are available for cosmetic injection in the United States. RimaBoNT-B has a demonstrably shorter half-life and is only FDA approved for treatment of cervical dystonia; its use is therefore typically limited to secondary nonresponders.[17–19] Comparing the efficacy of onaBoNT-A, aboBoNT-A, and incoBoNT-A is difficult because available head-to-head trials have enrolled relatively small numbers of subjects and are often industry sponsored. On the whole, these products have more similarities than differences; variations in potency, speed of onset, therapeutic duration, and immunogenicity are relatively minor when compared with BoNT-B.[20] Important factors in product selection, therefore, include physician comfort and familiarity with the product being injected, as well as patient preference and history.

The units used to measure different formulations of BoNT are not directly interchangeable. This designation is shorthand for "mouse unit," or the median intraperitoneal dose of toxin that results in death of a laboratory mouse (LD50).[21] Because each manufacturer uses a slightly different protocol, a corrective factor often has to be employed when a physician familiar with injecting one product switches to another. Fortunately, relatively reliable consensus nomograms have now been established for all available products. Units of onaBoNT-A and incoBoNT-A are generally interchanged in a 1:1 ratio, whereas 2.5 to 3 times the number of units are generally required for aboBoNT-A, and 40 to 50 times the number of units for rimaBoNT-B.

Cosmetic onabotulinumtoxinA (Botox, Allergan, Inc) was approved for the treatment of moderate-to-severe glabellar rhytids in 2002 and then became the first neurotoxin FDA approved for the correction of lateral canthal lines in 2013. It is available in 50- and 100-unit vials, and has a stable shelf life of 3 years at 2°C to 8°C.[11] According to the manufacturer, it should be stored at 2°C to 8°C after reconstitution and used within 24 hours. The package insert recommends dilution of 100 units in 2.5 mL of normal saline (40 U/mL). Some injectors prefer to use higher concentrations ($\leq$100 U/mL) in areas where there is a more significant risk of side effects from diffusion, and lesser concentrations (20–25 U/mL) for areas, such as the forehead, where more diffusion may produce a 'softer' look.[8] In 1997, the Botox formula was altered to reduce the concentration of complexing proteins; product immunogenicity has decreased measurably since this change was made.[22]

IncobotulinumtoxinA (Xeomin, Merz Pharmaceuticals, L.L.C.) was approved by the FDA for the treatment of moderate-to-severe glabellar rhytids in 2011. It is also available in 50- and 100-unit vials. According to the manufacturer, unreconstituted product is stable for 3 years at temperatures ranging from –20°C to 25°C. Independent studies suggest that the shelf life may be up to 4 years at room temperature.[23,24] It is shipped without dry ice, and can be transported between offices without refrigeration. Once reconstituted, it is certified as stable for 24 hours at 2°C to 8°C. Most practitioners use the same dilutions and dosing as for onaBoNT-A.[12,25] A variety of industry-sponsored noninferiority trials also suggest comparable onset of action and duration compared with onaBoNT-A.[26,27] The principal advantage of incoBoNT-A seems to be the absence of complexing proteins, which theoretically reduces the risk of immunogenicity and secondary nonresponse.[28,29]

AbobotulinumtoxinA (Dysport, Galderma Laboratories, L.P.) was FDA approved for the treatment of moderate-to-severe glabellar rhytids in 2009 and comes in 300-unit vials. The reported shelf life is 2 years.[11] It is shipped on dry ice and should be stored at 2°C to 8°C until used.[8] The manufacturer recommends that it be injected within 4 hours of reconstitution. The 300-unit vial is typically diluted in between 1.5 and 3 mL of sodium chloride (yielding a concentration of 100–200 U/mL). The majority of practitioners inject 2.5 to 3 units of aboBoNT-A for every 1 unit of onaBoNT-A or incoBoNT-A.[22] The main consensus observation regarding aboBoNT-A is that onset tends to be slightly more rapid, but duration of action is slightly shorter when compared with other BoNT-A formulations.[9,30] Some data suggest that aboBoNT-A may diffuse slightly more than other comparably diluted products, although this has not been linked to a higher incidence of adverse effects.[22] It is also important to know that aboBoNT-A may contain trace amounts of cow's milk protein because it is manufactured with lactose, and patients with true allergy (vs intolerance) should not be injected.

RimabotulinumtoxinB (Myobloc, Solstice Neurosciences, Inc) was FDA approved for cervical dystonia, and has not subsequently been extended to any cosmetic indications. In contrast with all BoNT-A formulations, it comes as a ready-to-use sterile liquid with an unrefrigerated shelf life of 9 months and a refrigerated life of up to 4 years.[31,32] Owing to its acidic nature (pH 5.6), injections tend to be more uncomfortable.[12] It also has a faster onset and considerably shorter average duration of efficacy (generally 6–10 weeks).[19,33,34] Because of this, cosmetic use is typically limited to rare secondary nonresponders who have developed neutralizing antibodies to BoNT-A.[12] Similar reductions in the concentration of complexing proteins have been achieved owing to refinements in the manufacturing process, and the rates of immune-related failure for cervical dystonia (which requires very high doses of neurotoxin) have fallen from 5% to 17% to 1.2%.[35,36]

Reconstitution, Handling, and Storage

All BoNT-A formulations are delivered as lyophilized powder in a vacuum-sealed vial. We draw up the chosen diluent in a sterile 3-mL syringe with a blunt cannula or large filter tip needle, which is then used to pierce the rubber stopper of the vial after it is cleaned with an alcohol pad. The vacuum should draw in the majority of diluent automatically, and mild pressure can be used to inject the remaining saline as needed (**Fig. 1**). We then roll the vial

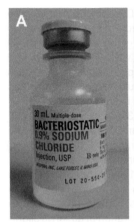
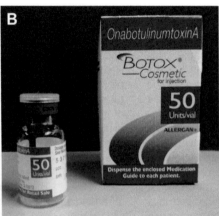
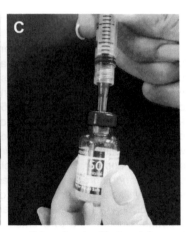

Fig. 1. (A) Preserved normal saline contains 0.9% benzyl alcohol, which has a mild analgesic effect and does not seem to compromise the potency or longevity of neurotoxin. (B) Representative 50-U vial of Botox. Note that the narrower neck of the 50-U vial is still broad enough to accommodate a 0.3-mL Ultrafine II Diabetic syringe. (C) The vacuum should draw in the majority of diluent automatically, and mild pressure can be used to inject the remaining saline as needed. (*Courtesy of* Allergan, Inc, Irvine, CA, with permission.)

gently to dissolve the product, taking care not to agitate it or cause foam to develop. Despite recent studies demonstrating that rough handling and agitation may not affect toxin potency to the degree once feared, we still believe it prudent to exercise caution.[37,38] In the case of incoBoNT-A, Merz Pharmaceuticals recommends that the vial be inverted to ensure that any leftover product under the cap is dissolved, and we commonly perform this maneuver for all toxins during reconstitution. Exposure of product to direct sunlight should also be avoided.

We then remove the metal cap and stopper from the vial using a household can opener or large Webster needle holder. This obviates the need to draw up and inject with separate needles. Even with smaller 50-mL vials, it is possible to obtain product directly with 31-gauge diabetic syringes, although care should be taken not to blunt the tip on the bottom of the glass container. Use of a hubless syringe with an attached needle minimizes waste. The vial can later be sealed with the rubber stopper if there is residual product to refrigerate.

All manufacturers recommend reconstitution with preservative-free sterile saline, but a 2004 consensus panel stated that preserved saline is the preferred diluent for the reconstitution of neurotoxins.[39] It contains 0.9% benzyl alcohol, which has a mild analgesic effect and does not seem to compromise the potency or longevity of the toxin (see Fig. 1A).[40,41] A number of authors have demonstrated that BoNT-A can be reconstituted with 1% or 2% lidocaine with epinephrine, but we have not found this to be necessary.[42,43]

All neurotoxin vials are labeled and marketed for single use, and injection is recommended within 4 to 24 hours. Despite this, the majority of clinicians store product that has been reconstituted for significantly longer periods of time. The current consensus is that product refrigerated at 2°C to 8°C for up to 6 weeks remains safe and effective.[44–46] There is some evidence that product may be frozen for up to 6 months without an appreciable impact on potency.[47] All cooled solutions, however, should be allowed time to equilibrate to room temperature to prevent injection site discomfort.[5] Regardless of the product, it is recommended that, after reconstitution, the solution be refrigerated rather than left at room temperature.

Product Dilution

Different physicians prefer a variety of toxin concentrations, and may even modify the dilution based on the location of injection. In general, more concentrated product has less risk of diffusion and may last longer, but some injectors prefer the 'softer' look that is achieved with higher diluent volumes in the forehead and lateral canthal region.[13,45,48] There are conflicting data regarding the extent to which greater diffusion with higher diluent volumes may predispose to additional complications. Carruthers and colleagues injected 10, 20, 33.3, or 100 U/mL of onaBoNT-A in the glabella (20 patients per group) and found no difference in therapeutic success or complications, although all 6 cases of eyebrow ptosis developed in the groups receiving more dilute injections.[49]

We have found the use of a 50 U/mL concentration for both onaBoNT-A and incoBoNT-A to be a simple and effective compromise for all of our periocular injections. Using this dilution, a 0.3-mL Ultrafine II Diabetic syringe (Becton Dickenson, Franklin Lakes, NJ) holds 15 units; 0.1 mL contains 5 units, and 0.05 mL contains 2.5 units. Using multiples of 5 and 2.5 makes calculating and injecting easy, and is convenient not to have to draw up 2 different concentrations for the forehead and glabella.

PATIENT PREPARATION AND POSITIONING

Contraindications to cosmetic neurotoxin injection are rare, but must be considered in all patients. BoNT is a category C medication in pregnancy and lactation, and it is prudent to avoid elective treatment. Neuromuscular disorders such as myasthenia gravis, Eaton-Lambert syndrome and amyotrophic lateral sclerosis can theoretically be worsened by neurotoxin injections.[45] Neurotoxins should be administered with caution in patients taking medications, such as aminoglycosides, tetracyclines, polymixins, penicillamine, anticholinesterases, and calcium channel blockers, that can theoretically alter conduction at the neuromuscular junction.[7,45] Hypersensitivity to any known constituent of the formulation (eg, milk protein with Dysport) is also a contraindication.[7]

Zoster reactivation has been described after neurotoxin injections as a rare side effect.[50] We typically reserve prophylactic acyclovir or valacyclovir, however, for patients with known cold sores or other herpetic manifestations, who are undergoing simultaneous treatment with other injectables or lasers.

We use alcohol pads to remove facial oils and makeup from the injection sites. In our practices, chlorhexidine scrubs are used in patients who are undergoing simultaneous dermal filler injections, owing to the higher risk of infection with atypical mycobacteria and the chance of developing biofilms. We rarely find it necessary to apply topical anesthetics such as EMLA (Astra Pharmaceuticals, Westborough, MA) before injection or to add analgesics apart from preserved sterile saline and occasional ice packs.

The patient should be seated upright with his or her head firmly supported by a headrest and at the injector's shoulder height.[8] The nondominant hand should be used actively to pinch up and protect various parts of the periocular and midfacial anatomy. Particularly in the glabellar region, pinching the corrugators protects the orbital rim and decreases the chance of toxin diffusing into the levator aponeurosis, which can result in blepharoptosis.

PROCEDURAL APPROACH
Forehead

The frontalis muscle originates from the galea aponeurotica, and inserts inferiorly onto the frontal bone and brow complex, interdigitating with the brow depressors. Twin bellies of the frontalis are often divided by a central tendinous aponeurosis. In patients where there is lack of movement between the lobes with forehead animation, some injectors elect to forgo central injection.[48] It is not necessary to inject lateral to the temporal fusion lines, because the frontalis muscle does not generally extend past this landmark. One can palpate these bony ridges in most patients, which emanate superiorly from the zygomatic process of the frontal bone at the superolateral orbital rim.[48] Careful attention should be given to the height and shape of each patient's hairline. Those with laterally receding hairlines may peak visibly, and often require additional injections in the lateral pretrichial region.

We typically do not recommend injecting below the midline of the forehead, because residual animation of the inferior frontalis muscle is necessary to prevent brow ptosis in many patients, even when the brow depressors are simultaneously injected. Others suggest staying at least 2 to 3 cm (or 1 to 2 finger breadths) above the orbital rim.[13,48,51,52] We recommend 2 to 2.5 units per site, with between 4 and 6 horizontally placed injections, depending on the width of the forehead. In Asian patients, more conservative dosing with 1 unit per injection site may be warranted.[53] In patients with longer foreheads, it is advisable to place additional injections superiorly, with a distribution pattern to be determined by the shape of the hairline. Some injectors have recommended a V-shaped configuration starting 2 cm above the medial brow and diverging superolaterally, but we have not found this to be the ideal distribution.[48] Injections may be intramuscular or subcutaneous, depending on injector preference, and have equivalent efficacy in split face studies (**Figs. 2** and **3A**).[54] Total dosing typically varies between 10 and 25 units, with male patients possibly requiring higher doses owing to greater muscle mass.[12,17,48]

There are instances in which frontalis injections should be avoided altogether, such as in patients who rely heavily on this muscle contraction: those with significant brow ptosis, blepharoptosis, or dermatochalasis, and some Asians with particularly heavy lids.

Glabella

The glabellar region contains the medial brow depressors, which include the corrugator supercilii, procerus, variably present depressor supercilii,

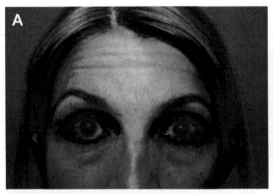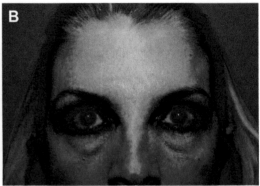

Fig. 2. (*A*) After injection of the forehead, maximum elevation of the forehead still produces gentle horizontal rhytids. We prefer to avoid overly aggressive injection with the goal of eliminating all movement. (*B*) Excellent cosmetic result in the same patient.

and superomedial orbicularis muscle fibers. The corrugators arise from the nasal process of the frontal bone, and extend to insert on mid brow skin near the supraorbital notch. Repetitive contraction in this area produces characteristic paired vertical rhytids (the "11s"). The vertically oriented procerus and flanking depressor supercilii muscles arise over the bony nasal bridge and insert on skin in the lower forehead between the eyebrows. Contraction produces horizontal glabellar lines. Prominent glabellar rhytids can unintentionally project anger, worry, or advancing age.[7,55] Injection of this region was the only FDA-approved indication for cosmetic BoNT up until 2013, and remains the most commonly performed neurotoxin procedure.[48]

Glabellar injections must be carefully delivered to prevent inadvertent diffusion and resulting blepharoptosis. Accordingly, the orbital rim should be protected with the nondominant hand and the injections should be placed no closer than 1 cm to the orbital rim and directed into the muscle bellies (see **Fig. 3**B, C).[7,8,45] A V-shaped pattern with 3 or 5 points is typically used.[14] The central injection is into the procerus, whereas the others are into the body of the corrugator supercilii muscles. The most lateral injection points are only needed in those with large, heavy corrugators.

We recommend 4 to 5 units per injection for the central 3 sites, and occasionally use supplemental injections of 2 to 5 units each if further lateral administration is desirable. We recommend pinching up the corrugator with the nondominant forefinger and thumb while using the thumb to apply pressure over the orbital rim.[13] The needle should not be directed toward the globe or eyelid, but rather at a slightly upward angle. We pinch up the belly of the procerus at the root of the nose and inject it perpendicularly. We find that gentle massage in

the superolateral direction serves to disperse toxin to the intended distribution, although this practice is not endorsed universally.[45] Total injection doses typically vary from 8 to 40 units, with higher dosing for men, who tend to have stronger medial brow depressors (**Fig. 4**, Videos 1 and 2).[17,53]

Lateral Canthal Lines ("Crow's Feet")

The orbicularis oculi is a circumferentially oriented sphincter muscle; contraction with eye closure and animation of the midface therefore produces rhytids that emanate radially from the lateral canthal region. Injection should be in the subcutaneous plane, at least 1 cm lateral to the orbital rim and 1.5 cm lateral to the lateral canthus.[51,56] Because eyelid skin is the thinnest on the body and tightly adherent to the underlying orbicularis oculi, even an intradermal injection reaches the targeted muscle. Injection in this area is similar to administering a tuberculin test: very superficial needle placement produces a wheel of fluid beneath the skin. Not only will this improve the precision of the injection, but it will also help to minimize bruising. The needle should be stabilized and directed such that it will not inadvertently traumatize the eye if the patient moves his or her head suddenly (see **Fig. 3**D). Injection of small volumes of more highly concentrated BoNT-A also helps to reduce the risk of blepharoptosis, lower lid ectropion, and double vision (Video 3).

Doses of 7 to 30 units may be given, typically divided among 2 or 3 injection sites.[7,17,53] Depending on the pattern of rhytids, however, the total dose may be split among a greater number of sites. We typically inject 4 to 5 units at each of 3 sites, with the central injection point in the same horizontal plane as the lateral canthal angle.

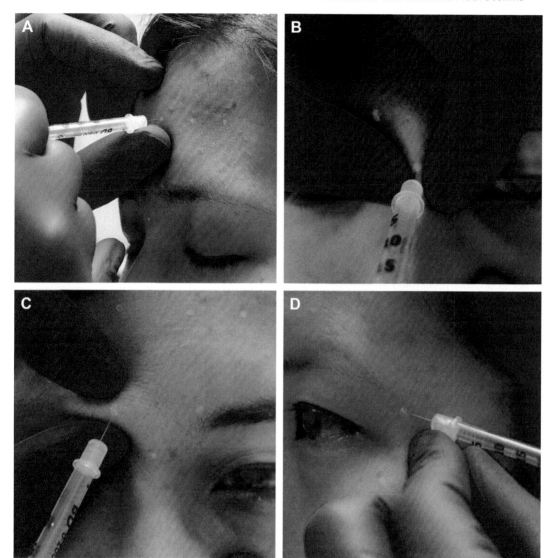

Fig. 3. (*A*) Technique for intramuscular injection of the forehead; note the avoidance of injection sites below the midline. (*B*) We pinch up the belly of the procerus at the root of the nose and inject it perpendicularly. (*C*) We recommend pinching up the corrugators with the nondominant forefinger and thumb while using the thumb to apply pressure over the orbital rim. (*D*) Intradermal injection of the crow's feet; the needle should be stabilized and directed such that it will not inadvertently traumatize the eye if the patient moves his or her head suddenly.

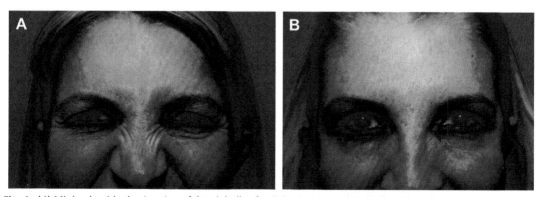

Fig. 4. (*A*) Minimal residual animation of the glabella after injection. Note that the lateral canthal and transverse nasal lines have not been injected; the 'bunny lines' are therefore prominent. (*B*) Resting appearance after glabellar injection.

Care should be taken not to inject too low over the malar eminence, because this can result in diffusion to the zygomaticus muscles, with concomitant upper lip ptosis. Additionally, injection nasal to the midpupillary line can lead to punctal ectropion and epiphora. It is wise to exercise caution in dry eye patients, because weakening the orbicularis oculi tone can exacerbate symptoms.

Infralid Injections

Some patients who perceive that they have "small eyes" desire enlargement of the vertical palpebral aperture for a "rounder" and more open appearance.[48,57,58] This can be accomplished with injection of the inferior pretarsal orbicularis, but such treatments must be approached with caution, so as not to unmask preexisting lower eyelid laxity. It is important to perform a "snap test" before injection. This test entails distracting the lower lid from the globe with the thumb and forefinger and letting it snap back. If the lid does not immediately reposition appropriately, infralid injections should not be contemplated. In general, they are contraindicated in older individuals, those with prior eyelid surgery, and patients with significant malar hypoplasia (the "negative vector" face).

One to 2.5 units may be injected subcutaneously, approximately 2 mm below the ciliary margin in the midpupillary axis.[57] In many Asian patients, the recommendation is to inject 1 cm below the ciliary margin, so as to preserve the appearance of the "jelly roll," but this may cause a puffy appearance of the lower lid owing to bulging of the central fat pad if the orbital septum is attenuated.[53] In patients who prefer to soften this jelly roll, 2 injections of 4 to 5 units each along the pretarsal orbicularis can be given to relax this muscle.

Transverse Nasal Rhytids ("Bunny Lines")

Obliquely directed rhytids on the nasal sidewall known as "bunny lines" may be seen with animation of the periocular region, and are particularly prominent in patients who have had prior neurotoxin injections in the glabellar region. They result from contraction of the transverse portion of nasalis muscle.[7,48] Between 1 and 5 units can be injected per side, taking care to avoid the angular vessels.[7,48] The pulse of the angular artery is typically palpable, and should be checked if there are any concerns regarding injection location. It is also important to avoid injecting too low in the nasofacial sulcus to avoid weakening the levator labii superioris, levator labii superioris alaeque nasi, and inferomedial orbicularis oculi (which will disrupt the "lacrimal pump").[48]

Brow Sculpting

BoNT injections can be used strategically to elevate and sculpt the brows by taking advantage of the fact that resting position is partially dictated by the balance between muscles that act as depressors versus elevators. Medially, the glabellar muscles (corrugator supercilii, procerus, depressor supercilii, and superomedial orbicularis oculi) all act as depressors. So long as these are injected preferentially to the lone elevator (the inferior frontalis muscle), 1 to 2 mm of medial brow elevation typically can be achieved.[7,13,49] The superior orbicularis muscle also can be injected immediately beneath the desired peak of the brow for an additional 1 to 2 mm of lateral elevation. This injection should be placed above the orbital rim, which is shielded with the thumb of the nondominant hand as the needle is directed superiorly (**Fig. 5**). However, injecting too high— into the region of the brow where the orbicularis oculi and frontalis interdigitate, or worse yet, into the inferior frontalis muscle—results either in no net effect or in brow ptosis. Between 1 and 6 units of concentrated BoNT-A may be injected.[59]

POTENTIAL COMPLICATIONS AND MANAGEMENT

Bruising, swelling, and hematoma formation owing to disruption of the dermal vascular plexus are

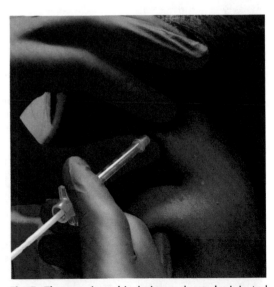

Fig. 5. The superior orbicularis muscle can be injected immediately beneath the desired peak of the brow for an additional 1 to 2 mm of lateral elevation. This injection should be placed above the orbital rim, which is shielded with the thumb of the nondominant hand as the needle is directed superiorly.

among the most common complications of neuro-toxin injection.[3,12,15,55] Fortunately, they are typi-cally mild and transient. Some injectors attempt to reduce the risk of bleeding complications by in-jecting in the subcutaneous plane for all sites except the corrugators and procerus. More concentrated toxin also reduces the total injected volume, which can be helpful to limit immediate postprocedure swelling. Although injections are not truly contraindicated in patients on anticoagu-lants, they should be counseled regarding the increased risk of hematoma formation and the benefits of stopping these medications 7 to 10 days before injection.[13] Management is with direct pressure and application of ice packs to encourage vasoconstriction. Although formula-tions of arnica are marketed to postinjection pa-tients, we do not typically recommend them unless simultaneous cosmetic surgery or use of dermal fillers is planned.

Injection site pain is generally limited and can be minimized with the use of a 30- or 32-gauge nee-dle. We routinely reconstitute with preserved ster-ile saline containing benzyl alcohol, but have not found it necessary to use lidocaine or EMLA cream unless simultaneous dermal filler injection is planned. Under no circumstances should neuro-toxins be reconstituted with sterile water, because this is nonphysiologic and results in considerable injection site pain.

Postinjection headache and nasopharyngitis/flulike symptoms were no more common with neurotoxin than placebo in the majority of clinical trials.[60–62] Patients can be counseled regarding the possibility of developing these symptoms and instructed to use over-the-counter analgesics, such as acetaminophen, as needed.

Brow ptosis is a potential complication of fore-head and misdirected glabellar injections. Caution should be exercised in injecting patients with thick soft tissues and prominent horizontal rhytids; pre-serving inferior frontalis action in these patients is critical to preventing descent of the brow com-plex.[63] We generally do not suggest injecting below the midline of the forehead in such patients. Special caution must also be exercised in the Asian population. Owing to lower insertion of the levator aponeurosis and orbital septum, the prea-poneurotic fat pad typically descends over the tarsal plate, resulting in a thicker and heavier eyelid. Consequently, many Asians rely on the frontalis muscle to act as a secondary brow elevator. Forehead injections should therefore be conservative. Of note, 90% of individuals have some degree of brow asymmetry, and this should be pointed out preinjection so that it is not mistaken for a complication of treatment.[13]

Treatment of brow ptosis can be accomplished with injection of the brow depressors (corrugators, procerus, depressor supercilii, and superomedial orbicularis), if this has not already been done. Management is otherwise expectant.

Any injections in the periorbital area can lead theoretically to eyelid ptosis via permeation of the orbital septum and spread to the levator palpe-brae superioris muscle. In practice, this complica-tion is seen most commonly with injections to the glabella or superior orbicularis. It is also possible to unmask a preexisting ptosis by limiting the elevation of the brow elevators with forehead injections.[22] Symptoms can appear as soon as 48 hours and with a latency of up to 7 to 10 days after injection.[13,48] Rates are strongly linked to injector experience; the incidence of blepharopto-sis fell from 5.4% to 1% between the first and sec-ond phase III trials for aboBoNT-A.[44] The best strategy is prevention using impeccable tech-nique; all injections should be performed at least 1 cm above orbital rim and 1.5 cm lateral to the outer canthus.[15] We also recommend smaller diluent volumes in the periocular region, and shield the orbital rim with the nondominant thumb when injecting the corrugators or superior orbicularis. Treatment entails the use of topical apraclonidine 0.5% ophthalmic drops (Iopidine, Alcon Labora-tories, Inc, Fort Worth, TX) 3 times daily until the symptoms resolve. This alpha-2-adrenergic agonist stimulates the sympathetically innervated Muller's muscle, producing approximately 2 mm of eyelid elevation, but it can also cause allergic conjunctivitis.

In patients with eyelid laxity, it is possible to pre-cipitate lower eyelid retraction and ectropion with lateral canthal or pretarsal injections. These eyelid malpositions can result in ocular surface exposure and reflex hypersecretion of tears. Overzealous in-jection of the orbicularis oculi can also weaken lacrimal pump function, resulting in symptomatic tearing through impaired drainage. Conservative measures such as lubrication with artificial tears and eyelid taping are recommended.

Double vision from migration of toxin to the lateral and inferior rectus is rare but may occur with overzealous injection of the lateral canthal lines.[48] Management is with temporary occlusion of the misdirected eye during important activities such as driving.

Injection of the lateral canthal lines that are overly inferior, medial, or deep can result in droop-ing at the corner of the mouth owing to paralysis of the perioral elevators (levator labii superioris, leva-tor anguli oris, levator labii superioris alaeque nasi, and zygomaticus major/minor).[13,48] Management is expectant.

Distal spread with dysphagia or systemic botulism is a theoretic concern, but has not been reported with the injection sites and doses typically used in the mid face. Nevertheless, starting in 2009 the FDA mandated that all BoNT formulations carry a black box warning regarding the distant diffusion of toxin.[12]

Primary nonresponse to BoNT is exceptionally rare; inappropriate dosing and product degradation are far more likely explanations that should be ruled out.[8] Secondary nonresponse owing to immune sensitization is also unusual with cosmetic doses of neurotoxin, but must be considered in any patient with a declining clinical response.[64,65] Most neurotoxins represent a foreign protein load, and are theoretically able to trigger the development of blocking antibodies. New formulations with reduced quantities of complexing clostridial proteins, however, have dramatically reduced the incidence of this complication. Patients are 6 times less likely to develop blocking antibodies in response to the "new" Botox formula introduced in 1997, which reduced the accessory protein from 25 to 5 ng per 100 units.[65–67] Cross-reactivity seems to exist only among BoNT formulations of the same serotype. Thus, substitution of rimaBoNT-B can be considered in patients with blocking antibodies to any of the BoNT-A formulations used in cosmetic practice.[12]

Allergy to any component of each BoNT preparation is possible, but reported reactions are limited to rare rashes and granuloma formulation. There have been no reports of anaphylaxis after facial injection.[15]

BoNT preparations are formulated with human albumin, but fortunately there have been no reports in the literature of virus or prion transmission.

POSTPROCEDURAL CARE

Recommendations for postprocedure care are straightforward. Many practitioners counsel their patients to remain upright for 4 hours after treatment and to avoid manipulating the treated area by hand, with the thought that these precautions may reduce unwanted diffusion.[22,45,63] Others go so far as to ask the patient to contract the treated muscles in an attempt to encourage faster uptake toxin uptake at the neural endplates; we have not found this to be necessary.[13] In the authors' practices, the only activity limitation routinely given is to avoid face down massage for 24 hours.

The full onset of action generally occurs within 10 to 14 days of treatment.[68,69] Patients are therefore encouraged to follow-up in 2 weeks for photographs and as needed touch-ups. Supplemental

injection past 2 weeks is not recommended, because some patients may attempt to extend the treatment duration by taking advantage of a free touch-up policy. Follow-up for full repeat injection should be booked 3 to 4 months after treatment, depending on past response patterns.

REHABILITATION AND RECOVERY

One of the significant advantages of cosmetic BoNT injection compared with other interventions is that recovery is generally very rapid and there is no downtime. Once the wheals of neurotoxin have been absorbed (typically within 15 minutes), it is often difficult to tell that any intervention has been performed.

OUTCOMES

The outcomes of experienced injectors are generally excellent, and patient satisfaction is high, provided that appropriate counseling has been provided regarding the endpoints that can realistically be achieved with neurotoxins. It is important to honestly inform a patient when his or her goals would be better met by other treatments, such as dermal fillers, laser therapy, or rhytidectomy.

SUPPLEMENTARY DATA

Supplementary data related to this article can be found online at http://dx.doi.org/10.1016/j.fsc. 2015.01.010.

REFERENCES

1. Scott AB. Botulinum toxin injection into extraocular muscles as an alternative to strabismus surgery. Ophthalmology 1980;87:1044–9.
2. Carruthers JA, Carruthers JA. Treatment of glabellar frown lines with C. Botulinum A exotoxin. J Dermatol Surg Oncol 1992;18:17–21.
3. Keaney TC, Alster TS. Botulinum toxin in men: review of relevant anatomy and clinical trial data. Dermatol Surg 2013;39(10):1434–43.
4. American Society of Plastic Surgeons. 2013 Plastic surgery statistics report. Web. November 8, 2014.
5. Chen JJ, Dashtipour K. Abo-, inco-, ona-, and rima-botulinum toxins in clinical therapy: a primer. Pharmacotherapy 2013;33(3):304–18.
6. Dressler D, Benecke R. Pharmacology of therapeutic botulinum toxin preparations. Disabil Rehabil 2007;29:1761–8.
7. Feily A, Fallahi H, Zandian D, et al. A succinct review of botulinum toxin in dermatology; update of cosmetic and noncosmetic use. J Cosmet Dermatol 2011; 10(1):58–67.

8. Lorenc ZP, Kenkel JM, Fagien S, et al. IncobotulinumtoxinA in clinical literature. Aesthet Surg J 2013;33(1 Suppl):23S–34S.

9. Flynn TC. Botulinum toxin: examining duration of effect in facial aesthetic applications. Am J Clin Dermatol 2010;11(3):183–99.

10. Kukreja RV, Singh BR. Comparative role of neurotoxin-associated proteins in the structural stability and endopeptidase activity of botulinum neurotoxin complex A and E. Biochemistry 2007;46:14316–24.

11. Giacometti JN, Yen MT. Update on botulinum toxins in oculofacial plastic surgery. Int Ophthalmol Clin 2013;53(3):21–31.

12. Flynn TC. Advances in the use of botulinum neurotoxins in facial esthetics. J Cosmet Dermatol 2012; 11(1):42–50.

13. Klein AW. Contraindications and complications with the use of botulinum toxin. Clin Dermatol 2004; 22(1):66–75.

14. Rzany B, Ascher B, Fratila A, et al. Efficacy and safety of 3- and 5-injection patterns (30 and 50 U) of botulinum toxin A (Dysport) for the treatment of wrinkles in the glabella and the central forehead region. Arch Dermatol 2006;142(3):320–6.

15. Carruthers J, Carruthers A. Botulinum toxin in facial rejuvenation: an update. Dermatol Clin 2009;27(4): 417–25.

16. Dubina M, Tung R, Bolotin D, et al. Treatment of forehead/glabellar rhytide complex with combination botulinum toxin a and hyaluronic acid versus botulinum toxin A injection alone: a split-face, rater-blinded, randomized control trial. J Cosmet Dermatol 2013;12(4): 261–6.

17. Berbos ZJ, Lipham WJ. Update on botulinum toxin and dermal fillers. Curr Opin Ophthalmol 2010; 21(5):387–95.

18. Matarasso S. Complications of botulinum A exotoxin for hyperfunctional lines. Dermatol Surg 1998;24: 1249–54.

19. Spencer JM, Gordon M, Goldberg DJ. Botulinum B treatment of the glabellar and frontalis regions: a dose response analysis. J Cosmet Laser Ther 2002; 4:19–23.

20. Bonaparte JP, Ellis D, Quinn JG, et al. A comparative assessment of three formulations of botulinum toxin A for facial rhytides: a systematic review and meta-analyses. Syst Rev 2013;2:40.

21. Adler S, Bicker G, Bigalke H, et al. The current scientific and legal status of alternative methods to the LD50 test for botulinum neurotoxin potency testing. Altern Lab Anim 2010;38:315–30.

22. Walker TJ, Dayan SH. Comparison and overview of currently available neurotoxins. J Clin Aesthet Dermatol 2014;7(2):31–9.

23. Grein S, Mander GJ, Taylor HV. Xeomin® is stable without refrigeration: complexing proteins are not required for stability of botulinum toxin type A preparations. Toxicon 2008;51:13.

24. Grein S, Mander GJ, Fink K. Stability of botulinum neurotoxin type A, devoid of complexing proteins. Botulinum J 2011;2(1):49–57.

25. Prager W, Huber-Vorländer J, Taufig AZ, et al. Botulinum toxin type A treatment to the upper face: retrospective analysis of daily practice. Clin Cosmet Investig Dermatol 2012;5:53–8.

26. Sattler G, Callander M, Grablowitz D, et al. Noninferiority of incobotulinumtoxinA, free from complexing proteins, compared with another botulinum toxin type A in the treatment of glabellar frown lines. Dermatol Surg 2010;36:2146–54.

27. Jost WH, Blumel J, Grafe S. Botulinum neurotoxin type A free of complexing proteins (XEOMIN) in focal dystonia. Drugs 2007;67:669–83.

28. Jankovic J. Botulinum toxin: clinical implications of antigenicity and immunoresistance. In: Brin MF, Jankovic J, Hallett M, editors. Scientific and therapeutic aspects of botulinum toxin. Philadelphia: Lippincott Williams & Wilkins; 2002. p. 409–15.

29. Lee JC, Yokota K, Arimitsu H, et al. Production of antineurotoxin antibody is enhanced by two subcomponents, HA1 and HA3b, of Clostridium botulinum type B 16S toxin-haemagglutinin. Microbiology 2005;151:3739–47.

30. Lowe P, Patnaik R, Lowe N. Comparison of two formulations of botulinum toxin type A for the treatment of glabellar lines: a double-blind, randomized study. J Am Acad Dermatol 2006;55(6):975–80.

31. Setler P. The biochemistry of botulinum toxin type B. Neurology 2000;55(Suppl 5):S22–8.

32. Trindade De Almeida AR, Secco LC, Carruthers A. Handling botulinum toxins: an updated literature review. Dermatol Surg 2011;37(11):1553–65.

33. Flynn TC, Clark RE II. Botulinum toxin type B (MYOBLOC) versus botulinum toxin type A (BOTOX) frontalis study: rate of onset and radius of diffusion. Dermatol Surg 2003;29:519–22 [discussion: 522].

34. Ramirez AL, Reeck J, Maas CS. Botulinum toxin type B (MyoBloc) in the management of hyperkinetic facial lines. Otolaryngol Head Neck Surg 2002;126: 459–67.

35. Dressler D, Hallett M. Immunological aspects of Botox, Dysport and Myobloc/NeuroBloc. Eur J Neurol 2006;13(Suppl 1):11–5.

36. Brin MF, Comella CL, Jankovic J, et al. Long-term treatment with botulinum toxin type A in cervical dystonia has low immunogenicity by mouse protection assay. Mov Disord 2008;23:1353–60.

37. Shome D, Nair AG, Kapoor R, et al. Botulinum toxin A: is it really a fragile molecule? Dermatol Surg 2010; 36:2106–10.

38. Kazim NA, Black EH. Botox: shaken, not stirred. Ophthal Plast Reconstr Surg 2008;24:10–2.

39. (Walker 25) Carruthers J, Fagien S, Matarasso SL. Consensus recommendations on the use of botulinum toxin Type A in facial aesthetics. Plast Reconstr Surg 2004;114(6Suppl):2S.

40. Alam M, Dover JS, Arndt KA. Pain associated with injection of botulinum A exotoxin reconstituted using isotonic sodium chloride with and without preservative: a double-blind, randomized controlled trial. Arch Dermatol 2002;138:510–4.

41. Sarifakioglu N, Sarifakioglu E. Evaluating effects of preservative-containing saline solution on pain perception during botulinum toxin type-a injections at different locations: a prospective, single-blinded, randomized controlled trial. Aesthetic Plast Surg 2005;29:113–5.

42. Gassner HG, Sherris DA. Addition of an anesthetic agent to enhance the predictability of the effects of botulinum toxin type A injections: a randomized controlled study. Mayo Clin Proc 2000;75:701–4.

43. Haubner F. Simultaneous injection of lidocaine improves predictability of effect of botulinum toxin. Laryngorhinootologie 2009;88:764.

44. Hexsel DM, De Almeida AT, Rutowitsch M, et al. Multicenter, double-blind study of the efficacy of injections with botulinum toxin type A reconstituted up to six consecutive weeks before application. Dermatol Surg 2003;29:523–9.

45. Tremaine AM, McCullough JL. Botulinum toxin type A for the management of glabellar rhytids. Clin Cosmet Investig Dermatol 2010;3:15–23.

46. Hui JI, Lee WW. Efficacy of fresh versus refrigerated botulinum toxin in the treatment of lateral periorbital rhytids. Ophthal Plast Reconstr Surg 2007;23(6):433–8.

47. Liu A, Carruthers A, Cohen JL, et al. Recommendations and current practices for the reconstitution and storage of botulinum toxin type A. J Am Acad Dermatol 2012;67:373–8.

48. Lehrer MS, Benedetto AV. Botulinum toxin - an update on its use in facial rejuvenation. J Cosmet Dermatol 2005;4(4):285–97.

49. Carruthers A, Carruthers J, Cohen J. Dilution volume of botulinum toxin type A for the treatment of glabellar rhytides: does it matter? Dermatol Surg 2007;33:S97–104.

50. Graber EM, Dover JS, Arndt KA. Two cases of herpes zoster appearing after botulinum toxin type A injections. J Clin Aesthet Dermatol 2011; 4(10):49–51.

51. Huang W, Rogashefsky AS, Foster JA. Browlift with botulinum toxin. Dermatol Surg 2000;26:55–60.

52. Frankel AS, Kamer FM. Chemical browlift. Arch Otolaryngol Head Neck Surg 1998;124:321–3.

53. Ahn BK, Kim YS, Kim HJ, et al. Consensus recommendations on the aesthetic usage of botulinum toxin type A in Asians. Dermatol Surg 2013;39(12): 1843–60.

54. Gordin EA, Luginbuhl AL, Ortlip T, et al. Subcutaneous vs. intramuscular botulinum toxin: split-face randomized study. JAMA Facial Plast Surg 2014;16(3): 193–8.

55. Monheit G, Carruthers A, Brandt F, et al. A randomized, double-blind, placebo-controlled study of botulinum toxin type A for the treatment of glabellar lines: determination of optimal dose. Dermatol Surg 2007;33(1 Spec No):S51–9.

56. Baumann L, Slezinger A, Vujevich J, et al. A double-blinded, randomized, placebo-controlled pilot study of the safety and efficacy of Myobloc (botulinum toxin type B)-purified neurotoxin complex for the treatment of crow's feet: a double-blinded, placebo-controlled trial. Dermatol Surg 2003;29: 508–15.

57. Flynn TC, Carruthers JA, Carruthers JA. Botulinum-A toxin treatment of the lower eyelid improves infraorbital rhytides and widens the eye. Dermatol Surg 2001;27:703–8.

58. Flynn TC, Carruthers JA, Carruthers JA, et al. Botulinum A toxin (BOTOX) in the lower eyelid: dosefinding study. Dermatol Surg 2003;29:943–50.

59. Cohen JL, Dayan SH. Botulinum toxin a in the treatment of dermatochalasis: an open-label, randomized, dose comparison study. J Drugs Dermatol 2006;5: 596–601.

60. Cavallini M, Cirillo P, Fundarò SP, et al. Safety of botulinum toxin A in aesthetic treatments: a systematic review of clinical studies. Dermatol Surg 2014; 40(5):525–36.

61. Carruthers J, Lowe N, Menter M, et al, Botox Glabellar Lines II Study Group. Double-blind, placebo-controlled study of the safety and efficacy of botulinum toxin type A for patients with glabellar lines. Plast Reconstr Surg 2003;112(4):1089–98.

62. Carruthers J, Lowe N, Menter M, et al. A multicenter, double-blind, randomized, placebo-controlled study of the efficacy and safety of botulinum toxin type A in the treatment of glabellar lines. J Am Acad Dermatol 2002;46(6):840–9.

63. Klein AW. Complications, adverse reactions, and insights with the use of botulinum toxin. Dermatol Surg 2003;29:549–56.

64. Torres S, Hamilton M, Sanches E, et al. Neutralizing antibodies to botulinum neurotoxin type A in aesthetic medicine: five case reports. Clin Cosmet Investig Dermatol 2013;7:11–7.

65. Naumann M, Boo LM, Ackerman AH, et al. Immunogenicity of botulinum toxins. J Neural Transm 2013; 120(2):275–90.

66. Aoki KR. A comparison of the safety margins of botulinum neurotoxin serotypes A, B, and F in mice. Toxicon 2001;39:1815–20.

67. Jankovic J, Vuong KD, Ahsan J. Comparison of efficacy and immunogenicity of original versus current

botulinum toxin cervical dystonia. Neurology 2003; 60:1186–8.

68. Nestor MS, Ablon GR. The frontalis activity measurement standard: a novel contralateral method for assessing botulinum neurotoxin type-A activity. J Drugs Dermatol 2011;10(9):968–72.

69. Nestor MS, Ablon GR. Comparing the clinical attributes of abobotulinumtoxinA and onabotulinumtoxinA utilizing a novel contralateral frontalis model and the frontalis activity measurement standard. J Drugs Dermatol 2011;10(10): 1148–57.

Avoiding and Managing Complications in the Periorbital Area and Midface

CrossMark

Satyen Undavia, MD[a], Donald B. Yoo, MD[a,b,c,d],
Paul S. Nassif, MD[b,c],*

KEYWORDS

• Periorbital complication • Midface complication • Lid retraction • Ptosis • Dry eye syndrome

KEY POINTS

• Most complications can be prevented by proper preoperative history and physical examination.
• A thorough understanding of the complex periorbital anatomy prevents inadvertent injury to crucial structures.
• Many complications can require conservative management with topical lubrication and waiting the appropriate time before performing any further intervention.
• Severe complications such as visual loss from orbital hemorrhage require prompt identification and treatment.
• Midface surgery is a safe and well-tolerated procedure, with most complications arising from imprecise implant, suture, or endotine placement.

INTRODUCTION

The eyes play a central role in the perception of facial beauty. The goal of periorbital rejuvenation surgery is to restore youthful proportions and focus attention on the eyes. This is validated by the public's interest in blepharoplasty, which is the third most common cosmetic procedure performed today, and for the foreseeable future.[1] Because of the attention placed on the periorbital region, the importance of preventing and managing complications in this area cannot be overstated. Critical to this concept is obtaining a thorough preoperative history and physical examination, which can reduce significantly the

incidence of many complications. This article focuses on the preoperative evaluation as it relates to preventable complications, followed by common intraoperative and postoperative complications and their management.

PREOPERATIVE EVALUATION FOR PERIORBITAL AND MIDFACE REJUVENATION SURGERY

After discussing the patient's goals of surgery, obtaining a comprehensive medical and surgical history is critical to preventing complications from periorbital and midface surgery. Patients should provide a detailed list of all prescription and

The authors have no disclosures.
[a] Head and Neck Associates, 301 West Chester Pike, Suite 101, Havertown, PA 19401, USA; [b] Facial Plastic Surgery, Nassif MD Plastic Surgery, 120 South Spalding Drive, Suite 315, Beverly Hills, CA 90212, USA; [c] Division of Facial Plastic and Reconstructive Surgery, Department of Otolaryngology - Head and Neck Surgery, University of Southern California - Keck School of Medicine, 1975 Zonal Avenue, Los Angeles, CA 90033, USA; [d] Division of Facial Plastic and Reconstructive Surgery, Department of Otolaryngology - Head and Neck Surgery, David Geffen School of Medicine at the University of California, 10833 Le Conte Avenue, Los Angeles, CA 90095, USA
* Corresponding author. Facial Plastic Surgery, Nassif MD Plastic Surgery, 120 South Spalding Drive, Suite 315, Beverly Hills, CA 90212.
E-mail address: drnassif@spaldingplasticsurgery.com

Facial Plast Surg Clin N Am 23 (2015) 257–268
http://dx.doi.org/10.1016/j.fsc.2015.01.011
1064-7406/15/$ – see front matter © 2015 Elsevier Inc. All rights reserved.

nonprescription medications, including topical eye drops. In additional to a general medical history evaluation, special attention should be placed on prior facial surgeries, history or symptoms of coagulopathies, prior anesthesia reactions, and conditions that may alter healing, such as diabetes and immunosuppression. Patients with systemic diseases such as Sjögren syndrome, rheumatoid arthritis, Grave's disease, or neuromuscular diseases should be evaluated appropriately and counseled regarding the increased risks.

Several aspects of the patient's history are specific to preventing complications of periorbital surgery. Keratoconjunctivitis sicca, or dry eye syndrome (DES) is a common condition that has a wide range of etiologies. Patients should be questioned regarding symptoms of dry eyes (redness, soreness, mucoid discharge changes), because blepharoplasty can both result in DES, or exacerbate the condition if present before surgery.[2] Prischmann and colleagues[3] reviewed 892 cases of both lower and upper blepharoplasty and evaluated the results of a dry eye questionnaire that was given to patients before and after their surgery. They found the incidence of DES and chemosis was 26.5% and 26.3%, respectively. Several variables also increased the incidence of both DES and chemosis, including concurrent upper and lower blepharoplasty, transcutaneous approaches, preoperative DES, preoperative skin laxity, male sex, and hormone therapy. They recommended that, in patients with increased risk factors, adjunctive lid tightening procedures should be performed to reduce the risk of this complication.

Korn and colleagues[4] reported on the correlation between laser in situ keratomileusis (LASIK) and blepharoplasty and found that all 6 patients in the study developed DES. Special precautions must be taken in these patients to prevent this complication.

During the preoperative evaluation, it is important to identity patients with Grave's disease. This condition is owing to autoimmune activity against thyroid-stimulating hormone receptors and is associated with orbital disease in 40% of patients.[5] It is characterized by glycosaminoglycan deposition, fibrosis of extraocular muscles, and adipogenesis in the orbit.[6] Patients suspected of having this condition should be evaluated by an appropriate specialist to manage and prevent medical complications. Although blepharoplasty is often required in the surgical management of this disease, there are often multiple stages and varying techniques to address the proptosis and lid retraction that are associated with this condition.[5,7]

A thorough periorbital examination is required before undertaking any operation to properly identify the anatomic structures contributing to the patient's complaints and to recognize features that can increase the risk of postoperative complications. Critical to maximizing outcomes after upper blepharoplasty is preoperative evaluation of the brow. Excessive contraction of the frontalis muscle occurs to compensate for significant upper lid dermatochalasia. If blepharoplasty is performed alone, relaxation of the brow will occur after surgery, which reduces the effectiveness of the operation (Fig. 1).[8] To properly identify brow ptosis, evaluate the patient in a relaxed gaze, or manually fixate the brow digitally while assessing for excess skin.

Failure to recognize upper eyelid ptosis results similarly in a dissatisfied patient. Ptosis is defined as a margin-to-reflex-1 distance of 2.5 mm or less. Proper preoperative examination and documentation is critical, because traditional upper blepharoplasty techniques alone does not address this condition adequately. In addition, ptosis is a potential complication of the surgery, and the etiology can be unclear if preoperative documentation omitted this physical examination finding.

Preoperative assessment of the upper eyelid crease is essential for incision planning. Unusually high creases can be a sign of levator dehiscence that, if present, should be addressed at the time of surgery. Lacrimal gland prolapse can masquerade as excessive fat, and injury to this structure can lead to postoperative complications such as DES (Fig. 2). The lacrimal gland is located laterally and intraoperatively has a pinkish color. If significant prolapse is present, this can

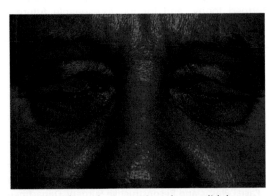

Fig. 1. Significant brow ptosis and upper lid dermatochalasia. Failure to address both problems will lead with suboptimal cosmetic and functional results. (*From* Massry GG. Managing the lateral canthus in the aesthetic patient. In: Massry GG, Murphy M, Azizzadeh BA, editors. Master techniques in blepharoplasty and periorbital rejuvenation. New York: Springer-USA; 2011. p. 185–98; with permission.)

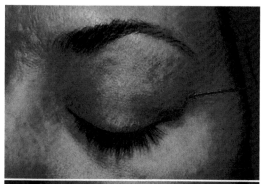

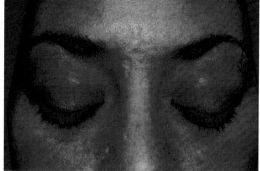

Fig. 2. Bilateral lateral upper lid fullness (*arrows*) classic for prolapsed lacrimal gland. (*Courtesy of* Guy G. Massry, MD, Beverly Hills, CA.)

be easily managed by pexying the gland to the orbital rim.

Proper evaluation of the lower lid helps to prevent complications from lower blepharoplasty such as ectropion/entropion, lid malposition, DES, and chemosis.[9] Horizontal lid laxity is measured by the snap test, in which traction is place on the lid and abruptly released (**Fig. 3**).

Prompt return to the globe indicates proper tone. The distraction test also measures lid laxity by maximally pulling the lid anteriorly. A distance of 6 to 8 mm indicates excessive lid laxity, which should be addressed by either lid tightening or shortening techniques. Malposition of the lower lid should also be assessed by placing upward traction on the lower lid. A normal lid should elevate to at least the midpupillary level. This evaluation is particularly important in revision cases.

Preoperative evaluation of excess skin in the lower eyelid is essential to prevent anterior lamellar shortening. This is evaluated by having the patient open their mouth widely while pinching the lower eyelid skin. If there is no excess in this position, removal of skin will put the patient as risk for lower lid malposition and ectropion.

A negative vector eyelid is described as a prominent globe with a recessed orbital rim/maxilla (**Fig. 4**).[10] Blepharoplasty in these patients is associated with higher complication rates, particularly lid malposition. The Hertel exophthalmeter measures the distance from the most anterior point of the lateral orbital rim and the anterior border of the globe.[11] The normal range for this test is 15 to 17 mm, with a range of 12 to 22 mm. For patients with significant exophthalmos, operative intervention should be modified by performing minimal fat excision or using spacer grafts to reduce the incidence of lid malposition. In addition, canthal-tightening procedures can exacerbate the malposition, as increased tension along the prominent globe will force the lid to retract further.[12]

Because of the many surgical options to manage facial rejuvenation of the midface, the challenge lies in the proper evaluation and

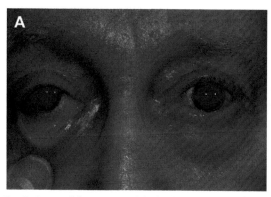

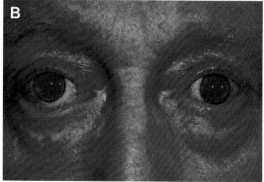

Fig. 3. Lower lid snap test. (*A*) The lid is distracted inferiorly. (*B*) The lid is released and allowed to return to its normal position without a blink. In this patient, the lower lid demonstrates laxity, because it does not return to normal position. (*From* Massry GG. Managing the lateral canthus in the aesthetic patient. In: Massry GG, Murphy M, Azizzadeh BA, editors. Master techniques in blepharoplasty and periorbital rejuvenation. New York: Springer-USA; 2011. p. 187; with permission.)

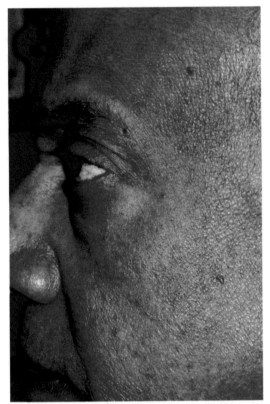

Fig. 4. Lateral view of a patient with a negative vector. The globe protrudes past the infraorbital rim. (*Courtesy of* Guy G. Massry, MD, Beverly Hills, CA.)

diagnosis of the specific anatomic changes that require correction. Patients should be questioned regarding prior history of midface trauma or rejuvenation techniques that have been utilized in the past. The entire lower-lid–cheek contour should be evaluated as a whole to maximize patient satisfaction. Evaluation and documentation of facial nerve function is important, because facial nerve injury is a potential complication. Patients with significant skin laxity and jowling are often better treated by rhytidectomy techniques either alone or in conjunction with midface lifting. Preoperative evaluation of the lateral canthus is also warranted; some authors have reported upward deflection after this surgery.[13]

COMPLICATIONS FROM UPPER AND LOWER BLEPHAROPLASTY

Meticulous preoperative evaluation and planning are essential to maximize patient outcomes and minimize complications. However, even the most adept and thoughtful surgeons will have complications in their practice. When complications do occur, the goal is to rapidly identify them and quickly initiate the proper treatment to minimize morbidity. Intraoperative and postoperative complications and their management are summarized (**Table 1**).

Intraoperative Complications

Corneal abrasions are a potential perioperative complication in any type of surgery. Inadvertent injury to the corneal epithelium can occur from oculotoxic sterilization chemicals, surgical instruments, gauze, or desiccation of the ocular surface. This complication is prevented by using corneal shields, which can be placed after applying tetracaine drops to the eye and a generous amount of petroleum-based lubricant. When corneal abrasions do occur, patients often complain of pain, foreign body sensation, burning, tearing, and blurry vision. Suspicion of this injury warrants prompt ophthalmologic evaluation with a fluorescein stain and a slit lamp. Management of these injuries depends on the severity, but most can be managed with 48 hours of topical erythromycin or bacitracin.[14] The surface can also be protected with application of contact lens.[15] Thermal injuries have been reported after cosmetic blepharoplasty and have resulted in postoperative astigamatism.[16] Treatment consists of topical antimicrobials followed by topical steroids to reduce scar tissue formation. Persistence of the astigmatism may require corrective astigmatic keratotomy.

Intraoperative and postoperative hemorrhage is a potentially devastating complication owing to the potential risk of blindness. Some degree of ecchymosis is expected after the procedure; therefore, a thorough clinical evaluation is necessary to correctly screen for those who require urgent intervention. Retrobulbar hemorrhage leads to a compartment syndrome, which puts significant pressure on the intraorbital contents. The exact mechanism of blindness from retrobulbar hemorrhage has been attributed to either central retinal artery compression or direct optic nerve injury. Mejia and colleagues[17] conducted a survey of 648 surgeons who performed 752,816 blepharoplasties, and found that the overall incidence of blindness from all causes was 0.0052%, and permanent blindness at 0.0033%. Hemorrhage can occur owing to vascular injury during injection, improper handling of orbital fat, and patient factors such as coagulopathies. Most instances occur within several hours after the procedure, but have also been reported several days after surgery.[18]

Retrobulbar hematoma presents with rock hard proptosis, chemosis, severe pain, and visual changes (**Fig. 5**). Ophthalmic consultation is

Table 1
Periorbital and Midface complication

Periorbital Complications	Cause	Prevention	Management
Dry eye syndrome	Missed preoperative, exposure, irritation	Preoperative history/examination, eye protection	Lubrication, lacrimal puncta ducts
Chemosis	Conjunctival irritation, disruption of lymphatics	Temporary tarsorrhaphy	Topical dexamethasone, topical phenylephrine, lubricants, conjunctivotomy and patching for severe cases
Ptosis	Missed preoperative, mechanical factors, levator injury	Preoperative history/examination, preserving levator	If persistent after 3 months, surgical ptosis repair
Diplopia/strabismus	Scar tissue, muscle injury	Limited deep cautery in lateral fat pad, muscle preservation	Local steroid injections, corrective strabismus surgery
Persistent dermatochalasia	Missed brow ptosis, underresection	Preoperative history/examination	Revision surgery, brow lift
Lower lid retraction/lagophthalmos	Muscle injury, preoperative lid laxity, anterior/posterior lamellar scarring, overzealous skin excision	Preoperative history/examination, canthal tightening procedures	Canthopexy/plasty, spacer graft, skin grafting, midface lifting
Corneal abrasion	Corneal exposure during surgery	Corneal protector	Lubrication, topical antibiotics
Hemorrhage	Anticoagulant use, vascular injury	Meticulous hemostasis	Surgical exploration, lateral canthotomy
Lacrimal gland injury	Missed preoperative, improper diagnosis	Proper identification intraoperatively	Lubrication
Infection	Surgical wound contamination, improper sterile technique	Perioperative antibiotics	Oral antibiotics, surgical decompression for abscess formation
Overcorrection	Inappropriate preoperative assessment	Thorough preoperative assessment, conservative fat removal	Postoperative fat grafting, fillers
Undercorrection	Inappropriate preoperative assessment	Thorough preoperative assessment, marking	Revision surgery
Midface			
Sensory nerve damage	Surgical error	Subperiosteal dissection	Expectant management
Facial nerve damage	Cautery, wrong plane of dissection	Subperiosteal dissection	Expectant management
Infection	Oral contamination	Copious irrigation, possibly avoiding intraoral route	Antibiotics, surgical drainage as indication
Asymmetry	Suture fixation	—	Revision surgery
Implant malposition	Improper placement, shifting	Tight subperiosteal pocket, implant fixation	Revision surgery

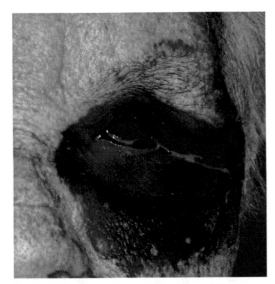

Fig. 5. Orbital hemorrhage. (*From* Massry GG. Managing the lateral canthus in the aesthetic patient. In: Massry GG, Murphy M, Azizzadeh BA, editors. Master techniques in blepharoplasty and periorbital rejuvenation. New York: Springer-USA; 2011. p. 112; with permission.)

requested early on in the course of therapy. Intraocular pressure is also elevated; however, surgical management is more dependent on the presence of visual changes. For patients with intact vision, conservative measures of cold compresses, intravenous osmotic agents, topical β-blocker drops, and acetazolamide are initiated. For patients with visual loss, aggressive management is required beginning with a lateral canthotomy. The wound should be opened to allow for decompression and washout. Any areas of active hemorrhage should be stopped with cautery. For patients with return of vision, they can be monitored closely and discharged with antibiotic prophylaxis and a tapered steroid dose pack. Persistent visual should be evaluated with an orbital CT. If a posterior hematoma is present, bony decompression is warranted.[18]

Postoperative Complications

Postoperative DES is a common complication after blepharoplasty, as mentioned. Proper preoperative evaluation is critical to limiting this complication. Postoperative lagophthalmos, orbicularis injury, and lacrimal gland injury can increase the risk of developing DES. Patients often complain of irritation, foreign body sensation, and blurry vision. Diagnosis is confirmed with a positive Schirmer test, in which filter paper measuring 35×5 mm is placed in a topically anesthetized eye. Less than 5 mm of wetness at

5 minutes is positive for DES.[19] The management generally entails usage of ocular lubricants such as artificial tears and a petroleum-based ointment. If symptoms persist, blockage of the lacrimal outflow via a punctal plug can be useful.

Chemosis often accompanies DES after blepharoplasty and is defined as swelling of the conjunctiva. It can be incited by inflammatory factors such as allergy or infection, as well as traumatic causes. After blepharoplasty, chemosis has been attributed to disruption of the lymphatic channels[20] or canthal disruption.[21] If significant chemosis is encountered intraoperatively, a temporary tarsorrhaphy should be performed to limit propagation of the chemosis and protect the conjunctiva. McCord and colleagues[20] described an algorithm for the management of postoperative chemosis. Conservative measures include topical phenylephrine, dexamethasone, and lubrication. Severe cases are managed with a conjunctivotomy and patching to apply pressure to the eye. Most cases resolve; however, symptoms can persist for several months despite treatment.

Lacrimal gland injury can occur during upper blepharoplasty, especially when the gland is prolapsed out of the orbit. The incidence of lacrimal gland prolapse has been reported to be as high as 60% in patients undergoing blepharoplasty.[22] The gland can be distinguished by its pink/gray color and its lateral location, where no fat pad is present in the upper eyelid. If identified intraoperatively, the gland should be preserved and repositioned into the lacrimal fossa by fixating the anterior margin of the gland to the arcus marginalis with an absorbable suture.

There are several causes for ptosis after upper blepharoplasty (**Fig. 6**). The most common is likely failure to properly identify ptosis before surgery. Injection of anesthetic agents causes a temporary ptosis if the levator superioris innervation is affected. Ptosis in the immediate postoperative period is usually owing to mechanical forces and

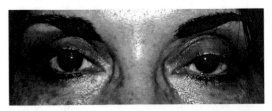

Fig. 6. Left-sided ptosis after upper blepharoplasty owing to levator injury. (*From* Czyz CN, Lam VB, Foster JA. Managing the lateral canthus in the aesthetic patient. In: Massry GG, Murphy M, Azizzadeh BA, editors. Master techniques in blepharoplasty and periorbital rejuvenation. New York: Springer-USA; 2011. p. 116; with permission.)

increased weight of the lid from edema. This edema resolves by 1 week after surgery as it is resorbed. Ptosis that persists months after surgery is likely owing to inadvertent injury to the levator aponeurosis.[23] The levator is more susceptible to injury at the inferior aspect of the lid where it attaches to the orbital septum and muscle to form the upper eyelid crease. To avoid injury, access to the orbital fat pads should be performed at the superior aspect of the lid through the orbital septum. The medial fat pad serves as an important landmark because it rests on top of the levator aponeurosis, preventing its injury.

Correction of ptosis requires operative exploration of the wound through an anterior approach. If a tear in the aponeurosis is identified, direct repair is performed. If the aponeurosis is disarticulated from the tarsal plate, it must be reattached using interrupted sutures.[24] It is helpful to perform this procedure under local anesthesia to properly assess the correction.

Lagophthalmos after upper blepharoplasty (**Fig. 7**) can occur owing to anterior lamellar deficiency (aggressive skin excision), incorporation of septal fibers into the skin during closure, or significant injury to the orbicularis muscle. Some degree of lagophthalmos is expected owing to upper eyelid edema and temporary orbicularis injury. For patients with significant lagophthalmos for greater than 2 weeks' duration, treatment should be considered to prevent exposure complications. Anterior lamellar shortening, which is diagnosed if pushing the brow inferiorly corrects the issues, can often be treated with full-thickness skin grafts. Septal adhesions should be explored early and lysed. A new technique that is gaining popularity is the application of fillers to correct lagophthalmos.[25,26] This technique has been used for patients with paralytic lagophthalmos[25] and for patients with superior sulcus syndrome[26] with excellent results.

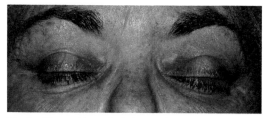

Fig. 7. Bilateral lagophthalmos after upper blepharoplasty. (*From* Czyz CN, Lam VB, Foster JA. Managing the lateral canthus in the aesthetic patient. In: Massry GG, Murphy M, Azizzadeh BA, editors. Master techniques in blepharoplasty and periorbital rejuvenation. New York: Springer-USA; 2011. p. 115; with permission.)

Infections after blepharoplasty are extremely rare, with most studies reporting a less than 1%[27,28] rate of infection. Infections typically occur 5 to 7 days after surgery and present with increasing edema, erythema, and pain. Infections can be classified as preseptal cellulitis or orbital cellulitis. Preseptal cellulitis is confined to the soft tissue superficial to the orbital septum and does not involve the orbit itself. Orbital cellulitis involves the orbit and is associated with proptosis, restricted extraocular muscle movement, and visual changes. Organisms involved in periorbital infections include beta hemolytic *Streptococcus* and *Staphylococcus aureus*. Most cases of preseptal cellulitis can be managed with topical and oral antibiotics and close follow-up. Orbital cellulitis requires more aggressive treatment, because visual impairment is a potential complication.[29] Patients should be admitted and receive intravenous antibiotics; imaging of the orbit is obtained. If there are any organized collections, surgical decompression is recommended. Possible approaches include upper blepharoplasty incisions, lateral orbitotomy, and endoscopic transnasal decompression for medial collections. Necrotizing fasciitis has been reported after blepharoplasty,[30,31] which presents similarly to other periorbital infections but has rapid progression and extends beyond the periorbital area. Fastidious and rapid diagnosis with surgical debridement can result in acceptable outcomes.[30]

Diplopia after upper or lower blepharoplasty may be temporary or permanent. It is thought to relate to direct trauma to the extraocular muscles during the procedure[32] or scar tissue formation, which limits extraocular muscle movement.[33] Syniuta and colleagues[32] looked at 12 patients who had strabismus after upper or lower blepharoplasty. Superior oblique injury was diagnosed in all 5 patients who had strabismus from upper blepharoplasty, and the rest had inferior rectus injury during lower blepharoplasty. Putterman[33] also reported 4 patients who had strabismus after lower blepharoplasty and found that all cases were owing to scar tissue formation in the lateral fat pad. This scarring was confirmed with MRI and treated successfully in 3 of 4 patients with systemic steroids and triamcinolone injections.

Diplopia has also been reported directly owing to lower lid fat repositioning.[34] In both of the reported cases, diplopia was present immediately after the procedure. One case was observed for 4 weeks and then explored surgically. Intraoperative findings showed scar tissue formation along the rim and arcus marginalis. Release of these bands resolved the diplopia. In the second case, the externalized Prolene suture used to reposition the fat was removed on postoperative day 2 and forced duction released the globe and returned the patient's normal gaze.

Postoperative crease and incisional issues are often related to preoperative assessment and markings. Canthal webbing can occur both medially and laterally after blepharoplasty (**Fig. 8**). The usual error is incision placement too medial or lateral, or too close to the lid margin. It can also occur from excessive anterior lamellar shortening. Mild cases can be first managed with gentle massage and steroid injections. For permanent deformities, surgical correction with V-Y advancement or multiple Z-plasties are performed. Massry[35] described 7 cases of lateral cicatricial canthal webs and 1 case of medial cicatricial canthal webbing. The lateral cases are managed with a V-Y advancement flap in combination with double Z-plasties with excellent results.

Poor scarring is a potential complication anytime the skin is incised. The upper eyelid skin is very forgiving; however, poor scar formation in this area leads to significant cosmetic deformity. Joshi and colleagues[36] looked at various closure techniques and found that a running 6-0 plain gut with several interrupted Prolenes resulting in the lowest rates of standing cone deformities and milia formation. Running locking 6-0 Prolene was associated with the highest rate of complications. Reexcision of the scar with meticulous closure techniques usually results in an acceptable outcome. For patients with track formation, subcuticular closure reduces the risk of recurrence. It is also critical to remove sutures 5 to 7 days after the procedure to reduce these complications.

The paradigm for the management of the periorbital fat pads has shifted from fat excision to fat repositioning and volume restoration. This maneuver is critical when trying to restore a youthful contour in this region and applies to both upper and lower blepharoplasty. The technique of fat repositioning has been well-established in lower blepharoplasty and can improve significantly the lower lid/cheek contour in patients with the classic double bubble deformity. Fat repositioning can be performed in the subperiosteal or preperiosteal plane with similar results; however, bleeding is slightly higher in the latter.[37] If hollowing does occur in the lower lid, this can be corrected with autologous fat grafting or placement of filler. Owing to the delicate quality of the lower lid, softer hyaluronic acid fillers are preferred to prevent palpable or visible abnormalities.

Hollowing in the upper lid is also a potential complication from overaggressive fat removal during upper blepharoplasty (**Fig. 9**). Not only does it result in a cosmetic deformity, severe cases can result in lagophthalmos.[26] Recent techniques have been described to prevent this deformity and involve limited removal of the central fat pad and repositioning of the nasal fat into the orbitoglabller groove.[38] Yoo and colleagues[38] described a technique in which the nasal fat pad is released and reshaped into a pedicled fat pad. The orbital rim is then exposed and limited subperiosteal dissection is performed in the area of maximal hollowing. The fat is then transposed into this hollow with a suture that is externalized over the skin. If hollowing does occur, hyaluronic acid fillers can be injected into the sulcus to correct the deformity as well.

Lower eyelid malposition is a challenging complication to manage (**Fig. 10**). Thorough preoperative evaluation can identify several factors

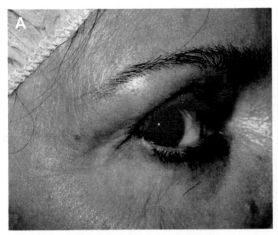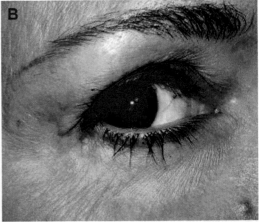

Fig. 8. Lateral canthal webbing after blepharoplasty before (*A*) and after (*B*) repair with combination of V-Y advancement and z-plasty. (*Courtesy of* Guy G. Massry, MD, Beverly Hills, CA.)

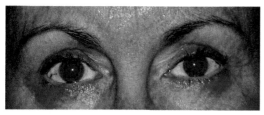

Fig. 9. Superior sulcus hallowing after overaggressive upper blepharoplasty. (*From* Czyz CN, Lam VB, Foster JA. Managing the lateral canthus in the aesthetic patient. In: Massry GG, Murphy M, Azizzadeh BA, editors. Master techniques in blepharoplasty and periorbital rejuvenation. New York: Springer-USA; 2011. p. 109–24; with permission.)

that predispose to this condition, as mentioned. There are different descriptors that fall under the category of lower lid malposition, including lower lid retraction, scleral show, ectropion, and entropion. When this complication occurs, patients are at risk for exposure keratopathies, significant irritation, cosmetic deformity, and blurry vision.

The lateral canthus should sit approximately 2 mm above the medial canthus and the lower lid should sit at the level of the inferior limbus. The lower lid is composed of 3 lamella: the anterior, middle, and posterior lamella. The anterior lamella is composed of skin and orbicularis oculi muscle, the middle of the orbital septum, and the posterior lamella of lower lid retractors and conjunctiva. Lower eyelid retraction can be caused by inadequate vertical laxity from lamellar shortening in 1 or a combination of the 3 lamella. To diagnose which of the 3 has the deficiency, cheek skin is pushed up to artificially recreate the anterior lamella. If the deformity is corrected, then the issue is from anterior lamellar shortening. If the retraction persists, middle or posterior lamellar shortening are more likely.

Vertical inadequacy results in ectropion with anterior lamellar shortening, entropion with

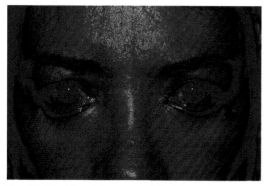

Fig. 10. Significant lower eyelid malposition 5 years after a skin muscle flap lower blepharoplasty. (*Courtesy of* Guy G. Massry, MD, Beverly Hills, CA.)

posterior lamellar shortening, and lower lid retraction with middle lamellar shortening. Ectropion, described as eversion of the lower lid away from the globe, most commonly occurs from excessive skin excision. A transcutaneous approach alone, without skin excisions leads to 2 to 3 mm of anterior lamellar shortening.[39] Correction of anterior lamellar shortening is traditionally done with full-thickness skin grafts. This technique can lead to scarring; however, if performed meticulously results can be acceptable even in cosmetic patients. The ideal skin donor is the upper eyelid skin owing to the thinness and color match. If patients have had recent upper eyelid surgery and this skin is not available, supraclavicular skin or postaurical skin is an option. One must thoroughly defat and debulk these grafts to maximize cosmesis.

Another option to correct lower lid malposition from anterior lamellar shortening is the midface lift. Repositioning of the suborbicularis oculi fat pad supports the lower lid, recruits skin and muscle, and rejuvenates the midface. Multiple approaches have been described, including a transconjunctival, temporal approach and subcilliary with subperiosteal or preperiosteal dissections. Marshak and colleagues[40] described a lateral canthal incision that allows for release of scar tissue and adequate access to the subperiosteal plane of the midface.

Middle and posterior lamellar shortening is managed with scar lysis and placement of a spacer grafts. Various autogenous and allogenic materials have been used with varied results. Common autogenous grafts include palate grafts, conchal cartilage, septal cartilage, temporalis fascia, and fascia lata.[41] Allogenic grafts, such as acellular dermis, have also been used; however, results have been less favorable. In 2003, Sullivan and colleagues[42] compared alloderm with palate grafts, and found a 57% contraction rate compared with 16% in the latter. Another option is described by Korn and colleagues[43] using dermis fat grafting. In their series of 11 patients, all showed significant improvement in lower lid malposition with symptomatic relief.

Another significant factor in lower eyelid malposition is horizontal lid laxity, which is assessed preoperatively with snap and distraction tests. If this laxity is present preoperatively, a prophylactic canthal tightening procedure can prevent lid malposition. Multiple techniques can be used to resuspend the canthus, including canthoplasty, tarsal strip removal, and canthal suspension. Canthal suspension is a technique in which a lateral canthal incision is made to expose the orbital rim. A double-armed suture is then passed through the lateral canthus and this suture is then anchored to the arcus marginalis in a manner that elevates and tightens the lower lid. The lid should be placed to create slight overcorrection, because some degree of laxity will recur.

MIDFACE

Midface rejuvenation can be accomplished using a multitude of different techniques and approaches. Each technique has its own set of advantages and disadvantages. It is important that, whichever technique is chosen, the surgeon understand the potential complications and their management (see **Table 1**).

Malar augmentation is a powerful technique that is generally well-tolerated. The most common approach is via an intraoral sublabial incision; however, implants can also be placed during lower eyelid blepharoplasty. Complications can be grouped into preventable and nonpreventable types.[44] Preventable complications include improper implant choice, migration, and improper placement. The proper size is one that is slightly smaller than the desired projection, because soft tissue over the implant increases the fullness.[45] Implant migration is the most common preventable complication. Creating a limited subperiosteal pocket to reduce mobility, placement of a temporary stay suture, or screw fixation of the implant can prevent this complication. There have been several reports of severe orbital complications from implant migration, including conjunctival extrusion, scleral erosion,[46] and intraorbital erosion.[47]

Several techniques have been described to identify the proper placement of malar implants.[44,48–51] Hinderer[48] describes 2 intersecting lines: one from the nasal ala to the tragus and the other from the oral commissure to the lateral canthus. The implant should be positioned in the superior lateral quadrant.

The most common nerve injured during malar augmentation with implants is the infraorbital nerve, owing to its close proximity of the dissection. These injuries are commonly transient[52] and resolve without intervention. Infection is also potential complication, as with any other surgical implants. These complications were reported in Proplast implants, and often occurred as a late sequela owing to maxillary sinus erosion.[53]

Transblepharoplasty approaches to midface rejuvenation can present with the same complications as those listed for lower blepharoplasty, including lid malposition with associated chemosis and DES. Hester and colleagues[54] reported a large series using this report and found that revision surgery was required in 19% of cases. Severe complication included persistent lower lid malposition despite canthoplasty procedures, which occurred in 3% of

patients. They attributed these complications to overzealous skin and muscle excision in patients with a negative orbital vector. In the same review, they also reported lateral orbital skin excess as a common complication, which was addressed by modified the incisions to include an upper lid approach, which allowed for more natural skin re-draping. They also emphasize the importance of preserving the middle lamella and preventing excessive injury to limit lower lid complications.

The transtemporal approach has been shown to be an effective technique to rejuvenate the midface. Because the lateral canthus and other orbital structures are not manipulated in this approach, lower lid malposition is not encountered.[55] The incision in the temporal tuft of hair carries a risk of alopecia, which can be limited by beveling the incisions to limit disruption of hair follicles. Bleeding and infection are not common complications. Abscess formation has been reported, which led to malar wasting requiring malar implants for correction.[56] The author of this series eliminated intraoral approaches to reduce this complication.

Maintaining the proper plane of dissection is critical to avoiding facial nerve damage. The frontal nerve crosses the zygomatic arch in the superficial temporal fascia. The incision posterior to the temporal hair is carried down to the superficial layer of the deep temporalis fascia. The dissection is continued in this plane toward the zygomatic arch, with the facial nerve above in the superficial temporal fascia. A temporal fat pad is encountered and then sharply entered. At this point, the plane of dissection is continued in a subperosteal plane for the remainder of the elevation. Temporary frontal nerve paresis has been reported as the most common complication in some series, occurring in 50% of patients.[57] Williams and colleagues[56] reported 3 cases of temporary frontal nerve injury and 1 case of buccal branch injury in a total of 325 cases. This same study had 1 case of permanent infraorbital nerve injury.

Alteration of the lateral canthal position was a potential complication owing to the vertical vector of pull performed during midface lifting. Kolstad and colleagues[13] looked at this outcome in 40 patients. They found that preserving a 2-cm area of the periosteum around the lateral canthus prevented this complication. Williams and colleagues[56] also found that canthal position was not significantly altered after midface lifting.

Endotine fixation has been purported by many to be a significant advancement in midface rejuvenation procedures.[57–59] The advantages include increased efficiency and accuracy of lift, decreased bunching, improved symmetry and decreased revisional rates.[57] Significant complications such implant extrusion or infection has not been reported.

SUMMARY

Surgeons, no matter how talented, cannot escape the reality that complications from surgery are inevitable. Once this has been acknowledged, it is the responsibility of the surgeon to take all measures to limit complications and have a thorough understanding of their management. Careful attention to the patient's concerns, history, and physical examination will help surgeons to avoid the majority of pitfalls that can occur from periorbital and midface surgery. In addition, a thorough understanding of the anatomy is crucial for all operative procedures. Finally, prompt recognition and management of complications, when they do occur, limit patient morbidity and provide the best chance to obtain excellent results.

REFERENCES

1. Broer PN, Levine SM, Juran S. Plastic surgery: quo vadis? Current trends and future projections of aesthetic plastic surgical procedures in the United States. Plast Reconstr Surg 2014;133(3):293–302.
2. Terella AM, Wang TD, Kim MM. Complications in periorbital surgery. Facial Plast Surg 2013;29(1): 64–70.
3. Prischmann J, Sufyan A, Ting JY, et al. Dry eye symptoms and chemosis following blepharoplasty: a 10-year retrospective review of 892 cases in a single-surgeon series. JAMA Facial Plast Surg 2013;15(1):39–46.
4. Korn BS, Kikkawa DO, Schanzlin DJ. Blepharoplasty in the post–laser in situ keratomileusis patient: preoperative considerations to avoid dry eye syndrome. Plast Reconstr Surg 2007;119(7): 2232–9.
5. Maheshwari R, Weis E. Thyroid associated orbitopathy. Indian J Ophthalmol 2012;60(2):87–93.
6. Bahn RS, Heufelder AE. Pathogenesis of graves' ophthalmopathy. N Engl J Med 1993;329:1468–75.
7. Hoenig JA. Comprehensive management of eyebrow and forehead ptosis. Otolaryngol Clin North Am 2005;38(5):947–84.
8. Hester TR Jr, Douglas T, Szczerba S. Decreasing complications in lower lid and midface rejuvenation: the importance of orbital morphology, horizontal lower lid laxity, history of previous surgery, and minimizing trauma to the orbital septum: a critical review of 269 consecutive cases. Plast Reconstr Surg 2009;123(3):1037–49.
9. Yokoi N, Komuro A, Nishii M, et al. Clinical impact of conjunctivochalasis on the ocular surface. Cornea 2005;24(8):S24–31.
10. Hirmand H, Codner MA, McCord CD, et al. Prominent eye: operative management of lower lid and midfacial rejuvenation and the morphologic classification system. Plast Reconstr Surg 2002;110:620.
11. Jelks GW, Jelks EB. Preoperative evaluation of the blepharoplasty patient. Bypassing the pitfalls. Clin Plast Surg 1993;20:213.
12. Glavas I. The diagnosis and management of blepharoplasty complications. Otolaryngol Clin North Am 2005;38:1009–21.
13. Kolstad CK, Quatela VC. A quantitative analysis of lateral canthal position following endoscopic forehead-midface–lift surgery. JAMA Facial Plast Surg 2013;15(5):352–7.
14. Segal KL, Fleischut PM, Kim C, et al. Evaluation and treatment of perioperative corneal abrasions. J Ophthalmol 2014;2014:901901.
15. Pullum KW, Whiting MA, Buckley RJ. Scleral contact lenses: the expanding role. Cornea 2005;24:269–77.
16. Chou B, Boxer Wachler BS. Astigmatism after corneal thermal injury. J Cataract Refract Surg 2001;27(5):784–6.
17. Mejia JD, Egro FM, Nahai F. Visual loss after blepharoplasty: incidence, management, and preventive measures. Aesthet Surg J 2011;31(1):21–9.
18. Teng CC, Reddy S, Wong JJ, et al. Retrobulbar hemorrhage nine days after cosmetic blepharoplasty resulting in permanent visual loss. Ophthal Plast Reconstr Surg 2006;22:388–9.
19. Kaštelan S, Tomić M, Salopek-Rabatić J, et al. Diagnostic procedures and management of dry eye. Biomed Res Int 2013;2013:1–6.
20. McCord CD, Kreymerman P, Nahai F, et al. Management of post blepharoplasty chemosis original. Aesthet Surg J 2013;33:654–61.
21. Maffi TR, Chang S, Friedland JA. Traditional lower blepharoplasty: additional support necessary? A 30-year review. Plast Reconstr Surg 2011;128:265–73.
22. Massry GG. Prevalence of lacrimal gland prolapse in the functional blepharoplasty population. Ophthal Plast Reconstr Surg 2011;27:410–3.
23. Baylis HI, Sutcliffe T, Fett DR. Levator injury during blepharoplasty. Arch Ophthalmol 1984;102(4):570–1.
24. Finsterer J, Vienna A. Ptosis: causes, presentation, and management. Aesthetic Plast Surg 2003;27: 193–204.
25. Mancini R, Taban M, Lowinger A, et al. Use of hyaluronic Acid gel in the management of paralytic lagophthalmos: the hyaluronic acid gel "gold weight". Ophthal Plast Reconstr Surg 2009;25(1):23–6.
26. Leyngold IM, Berbos ZJ, McCann JD, et al. Use of hyaluronic acid gel in the treatment of lagophthalmos in sunken superior sulcus syndrome. Ophthal Plast Reconstr Surg 2014;30(2):175–9.

27. Lee EW, Holtebeck AC, Harrison AR. Infection rates in outpatient eyelid surgery. Ophthal Plast Reconstr Surg 2009;25(2):109–10.

28. Carter SR, Stewart JM, Kahn J, et al. Infection after blepharoplasty with and without carbon dioxide laser resurfacing. Ophthalmology 2003;110:1430–2.

29. Juthani V, Zoumalan CI, Lisman RD, et al. Successful management of methicillin-resistant *Staphylococcus aureus* orbital cellulitis after blepharoplasty. Plast Reconstr Surg 2010;126(6):305–7.

30. Suñer IJ, Meldrum ML, Johnson TE, et al. Necrotizing fasciitis after cosmetic blepharoplasty. Am J Ophthalmol 1999;128(3):367–8.

31. Laouar K, Ruban JM, Baggio E, et al. Cosmetic blepharoplasty complicated by necrotizing periorbital fasciitis: a case report. J Fr Ophtalmol 2012; 35(6):437.e1–8.

32. Syniuta LA, Goldberg RA, Thacker NM, et al. Acquired strabismus following cosmetic blepharoplasty. Plast Reconstr Surg 2003;111(6):2053–9.

33. Putterman AM. Acquired strabismus following cosmetic blepharoplasty. Plast Reconstr Surg 2004;113(3):1069–70 [author reply: 1070–1].

34. Goldberg RA, Yuen VH. Restricted ocular movements following lower eyelid fat repositioning. Plast Reconstr Surg 2002;110(1):302–5 [discussion: 306–8].

35. Massry G. Cicatricial canthal webs. Ophthal Plast Reconstr Surg 2011;6:426–30.

36. Joshi AS, Janjanin S, Tanna N, et al. Does suture material and technique really matter? Lessons learned from 800 consecutive blepharoplasties. Laryngoscope 2007;117(6):981–4.

37. Yoo DB, Peng GL, Massry GG. Transconjunctival lower blepharoplasty with fat repositioning: a retrospective comparison of transposing fat to the subperiosteal vs supraperiosteal planes. JAMA Facial Plast Surg 2013;15(3):176–81.

38. Yoo DB, Peng GL, MAssry GG. Effacing the orbitoglabellar groove with transposed upper eyelid fat. Ophthal Plast Reconstr Surg 2013;29:220–4.

39. Kulwin DR, Kersten RC. Blepharoplasty and brow elevation. Ophthalmic plastic surgery: prevention and management of complications. New York: Raven Press; 1994. p. 91–111.

40. Marshak H, Morrow DM, Dresner SC. Small incision preperiosteal midface lift for correction of lower eyelid retraction. Ophthal Plast Reconstr Surg 2010;26(3):176–81.

41. Massry GG. Master techniques in blepharoplasty and periorbital rejuvenation. New York: Springer; 2011. Print.

42. Sullivan SA, Dailey RA. Graft contraction: a comparison of acellular dermis versus hard palate mucosa in lower eyelid surgery. Ophthal Plast Reconstr Surg 2003;19(1):14–24.

43. Korn BS, Kikkawa DO, Cohen SR, et al. Treatment of lower eyelid malposition with dermis fat grafting. Ophthalmology 2008;115(4):744–51.

44. Wilkinson TS. Complications in aesthetic malar augmentation. Plast Reconstr Surg 1983;71:643–7.

45. Constantinides MS, Galli SK, Miller PJ, et al. Malar, submalar, and midfacial implants. Facial Plast Surg 2000;16(1):35–44.

46. Menon V, Gupta H. An unusual complication of malar augmentation: transconjunctival exposure and scleral erosion. Ophthal Plast Reconstr Surg 2012; 28(1):7–9.

47. Hatten K, Morales RE, Wolf JS. Intraorbital erosion of a malar implant resulting in mastication-induced vision changes. Ear Nose Throat J 2012;91(11):23–5.

48. Hinderer UT. Malar implants for the improvement of facial appearance. Plast Reconstr Surg 1975;56: 157–65.

49. Silver WE. The use of alloplast material in contouring the face. Facial Plast Surg 1986;3:81–98.

50. Powell NB, Riley RW, Lamb DR. A new approach to evaluation and surgery of the malar complex. Ann Plast Surg 1988;20:206–14.

51. Prendergast M, Schoenrock LD. Malar augmentation. Arch Otolaryngol Head Neck Surg 1989;115: 964–9.

52. Metzinger SE, McCollough EG, Campbell JP, et al. Malar augmentation: a 5-year retrospective review of the silastic midfacial malar implant. Arch Otolaryngol Head Neck Surg 1999;125(9):980–7.

53. Adams JR, Kawamoto HK. Late infection following aesthetic malar augmentation with Proplast implants. Plast Reconstr Surg 1995;95:383–4.

54. Hester TR, Codner MA, McCord CD, et al. Evolution of technique of the direct transblepharoplasty approach for the correction of lower lid and midfacial aging: maximizing results and minimizing complications in a 5-year experience. Plast Reconstr Surg 2000;105(1):393–406.

55. Chaiet SR, Williams EF 3rd. Understanding midfacial rejuvenation in the 21st century. Facial Plast Surg 2013;29(1):40–5.

56. Williams EF, Vargas H, Dahiya R, et al. Midfacial rejuvenation via a minimal-incision brow-lift approach critical evaluation of a 5-year experience. Arch Facial Plast Surg 2003;5(6):470–8.

57. Saltz R, Ohana B. Thirteen years of experience with the endoscopic midface lift. Aesthet Surg J 2012; 32(8):927–36.

58. Hönig JF. Subperiosteal endotine-assisted vertical upper midface lift. Aesthet Surg J 2007;27(3): 276–88.

59. Berkowitz RL, Apfelberg DB, Simeon S. Midface lift technique with use of a biodegradable device for tissue elevation and fixation. Aesthet Surg J 2005; 25(4):376–82.

Index

Moving?

Make sure your subscription moves with you!

To notify us of your new address, find your **Clinics Account Number** (located on your mailing label above your name), and contact customer service at:

Email: journalscustomerservice-usa@elsevier.com

800-654-2452 (subscribers in the U.S. & Canada)
314-447-8871 (subscribers outside of the U.S. & Canada)

Fax number: 314-447-8029

Elsevier Health Sciences Division
Subscription Customer Service
3251 Riverport Lane
Maryland Heights, MO 63043

*To ensure uninterrupted delivery of your subscription, please notify us at least 4 weeks in advance of move.